Praise for *The Safety Playbook*

"As a proud CFO of a highly reputed healthcare organization, I remember it was hard to believe Dr. Byrnes's (or "John," as he prefers) claims of the safety crisis. Then I learned the data. And the cost associated. I quickly became motivated to join the safety improvement team. In this book, Dr. Byrnes, along with Susan Teman, provide practical guidance for healthcare professionals to also 'join the team.' It's a must-do agenda, and a must read."

Joseph J. Fifer, FHFMA, CPA
President and CEO
Healthcare Financial Management Association

"Once again, Dr. Byrnes has proven himself to be one of the foremost authorities on healthcare quality in the nation. This time, he, and coauthor Susan Teman, have focused on arguably the number one clinical imperative for hospitals: patient safety. As always, Dr. Byrnes and Ms. Teman present a practical approach to a complex issue."

Bruce P. Hagen
President
OhioHealth Marion General Hospital

"*The Safety Playbook* offers tangible, practical, and realistic approaches for how to refine patient safety in healthcare. This current era of patient safety is almost 20 years in evolution now, and we still are not as far along the trajectory as needed. This book clearly helps us move closer to the goal line—but that line keeps shifting, and we still need these tools to win the game. It's a must read!"

Peter Angood, MD
President and CEO
American Association for Physician Leadership

THE SAFETY PLAYBOOK

THE SAFETY PLAYBOOK

A Healthcare Leader's Guide to Building a High-Reliability Organization

John Byrnes and Susan Teman

Forewords by David B. Nash and Carson F. Dye

ACHE Management Series

Your board, staff, or clients may also benefit from this book's insight. For more information on quantity discounts, contact the Health Administration Press Marketing Manager at (312) 424-9450.

22 21 20 19 18 5 4 3 2 1

Library of Congress Cataloging-in-Publication Data

Names: Byrnes, John (Anesthesiologist), author.
Title: The safety playbook : a healthcare leader's guide to building a high-reliability organization / John Byrnes and Susan Teman.
Description: Chicago, IL : HAP, [2018] | Series: ACHE management series | Includes bibliographical references.
Identifiers: LCCN 2017039085 (print) | LCCN 2017043339 (ebook) | ISBN 9781567939460 (ebook) | ISBN 9781567939477 (xml) | ISBN 9781567939484 (epub) | ISBN 9781567939491 (mobi) | ISBN 9781567939453 (alk. paper)
Subjects: LCSH: Medical errors—Prevention. | Health services administration.
Classification: LCC R729.8 (ebook) | LCC R729.8 .B97 2018 (print) | DDC 610.28/9—dc23
LC record available at https://lccn.loc.gov/2017039085

The paper used in this publication meets the minimum requirements of American National Standard for Information Sciences—Permanence of Paper for Printed Library Materials, ANSI Z39.48-1984. ♾™

Acquisitions editor: Jennette McClain; Project manager: Joyce Dunne; Cover designer: Brad Norr; Layout: PerfecType

Found an error or a typo? We want to know! Please e-mail it to hapbooks@ache.org, mentioning the book's title and putting "Book Error" in the subject line.

For photocopying and copyright information, please contact Copyright Clearance Center at www.copyright.com or at (978) 750-8400.

Health Administration Press
A division of the Foundation of the American
College of Healthcare Executives
One North Franklin Street, Suite 1700
Chicago, IL 60606-3529
(312) 424-2800

To my wife, Lori, for her constant love, support, and encouragement in all things.
And to Mom and Dad for starting me on this path.
—John Byrnes

This book is dedicated to Dave, Ryan, Adam, and Emma. Because of you, I am brave.
—Susan Teman

Contents

Foreword

CAN LIGHTNING STRIKE the same location twice? Apparently so. John Byrnes, this time joined by his colleague Susan Teman, has done it again. Just two years ago, I had the privilege of writing the foreword to his previous book, *The Quality Playbook* (Second River Healthcare, 2015). Now John is back, publishing the companion "playbook" with Susan as coauthor and Health Administration Press as publisher.

Not only has literary lightning struck the same place twice, but this time John and Susan have given us one of the most tightly constructed, useful, and pragmatic texts in the field. I'm confident in this assessment, given the fact that I have written, edited, or contributed to seven such books in the past 30 years and have taught thousands of physicians and other leaders the fundamentals of quality and safety. Today, I'm proud to be the founding dean of the nation's first College of Population Health, where we offer a master's degree in healthcare quality and safety. I only wish this book had been available earlier so that previous students could have benefited from using it in our online classroom.

What stands out in my mind about *The Safety Playbook* are the specific, detailed instructions as to what to do immediately to reduce the epidemic of medical error. It's a playbook of instructions for saving lives. Why haven't others written comparable playbooks previously? It's a head scratcher, for sure.

Imagine being introduced to the essential concepts of high reliability without the typical turgid jargon that permeates our field. This book does just that. In addition, in an era characterized by "measurement madness," the text cuts right to the critical knowledge necessary for readers to not only grasp the safety field quickly but acquire the wherewithal to make a significant—and urgently needed—reduction in error rates in every sector described in the book.

In particular, two chapters resonate with me: chapter 9, focused on the role of the board in safety, and chapter 17, on simulation.

Having served on the board of two major not-for-profit delivery systems—Mercy Health in Cincinnati and Main Line Health in Philadelphia—in tandem for more than 18 years, I have a visceral appreciation for how important the board's role is in establishing a culture of safety. This is an often-overlooked area, and John and Susan gives it the kind of emphasis it deserves.

Reading chapter 17, on simulation, made me envious of current and upcoming trainees who have the opportunity to work in a simulation center and test their skills without real clinical consequences on a real patient. I'm convinced that simulation taking place both in situ and in a specialized center is an important tool in the toolkit that enables us to chisel away at the error rate in US healthcare delivery.

Part V, on communication, was my favorite of all seven parts comprising the book. The notion that intimidation in a work setting can kill is important; however, it rarely receives the kind of attention it deserves. Bringing the concept of the sterile cockpit from aviation to the healthcare delivery system was expertly handled by John and Susan. Also presented in part V is the simple safety practice of insisting that everyone on the team call one another by their first name. I wish I could have a nickel for every time I have told a junior colleague, nurse, physical therapist, respiratory therapist, or other team members to please call me "David."

The challenge brought to light by *The Safety Playbook* is how we, as a profession, will translate this wonderful gift into something that gets widely used on the front lines. Having been on the front lines of our movement for nearly 30 years, I am not sanguine that we have the political will to accomplish this critical goal. I'm heartened by the publication of *The Safety Playbook*, and I'm grateful to John and Susan for their scholarship. That said, I remain only cautiously optimistic that we can fulfill our sworn duty to reduce harm.

I know we will have achieved an important milestone when this outstanding book becomes required reading in every college of medicine and school of nursing throughout the country—I hope I am still around to see this happen. I am grateful to John and Susan for their important contribution, reflecting their own time on the front lines. For those who are coming up behind us, there is an important sense of hope for the future. The intended readers of *The Safety Playbook* have taken a sworn oath to reduce error. Let's make this book more than an amulet around the neck of our up-and-coming colleagues, and let's put its guidance into action as soon as we put the book down.

David B. Nash, MD, MBA
Dean, Jefferson College of Population Health

Foreword

The Safety Playbook. What reaction do those words inspire in you? Boring, humdrum, something for those who work at the bedside? Sigh. Yawn. Ugh. "I doubt this is a page turner. Do I really need to read this? Does it apply to me? Maybe I should just buy one for the members of the quality committee."

Or maybe this thought: "Hey, we're already a high-reliability organization (HRO); we don't need this. We already have it covered."

Now consider this: Medical errors are the third leading cause of death in the United States. Go ahead and quibble, argue that they are actually fifth or ninth. So what?

Well, so what? They cause death. I have no doubt that anyone who has personally experienced a medical error or near error will find this book convincing. And I have no doubt that the healthcare workers on the line for safety and quality will also find this book very helpful.

But I write this foreword in part not for them but for the "leaders" who do not find this book as compelling as one on finance, engaging physicians, or strategy. My personal interest is leadership—finding it, assessing it, recruiting it, developing it, working with it, and the individuals who practice it. My hope is that many leaders will see this book as an important part of their reading list. Yes, I hope they will buy copies for those on the front lines of patient safety and quality. And even though they may have already implemented HRO principles in their organizations, I hope they will add this to their body of knowledge. One good application would be to use the book as an audit tool, for example.

I have known John Byrnes for almost 20 years and Susan for about 2 years. Both are passionate about what they do. They are passionate first, and very competent second. Their offering is not a sermon or homily for us to "do better in safety and quality." They show us how to do it. They speak to the board, to the CEO, to the senior team, to the chief financial officer, to the clinicians. This is a readable book and one that will be used day after day by those at the battle lines, and it will certainly be read by those in the C-suite.

Leaders in our field have answered a calling. We are unique. We serve and we care for those in circumstances where they are at their most vulnerable. This description applies to all leaders, whether they work with clinicians or numbers or software or strategy. The very best leaders possess that internal value of caring—caring that their places of healing do not harm. Leaders: *Primum non nocere.* First, do no harm. Leaders at all levels must be constantly aware of and vigilant about how their actions and examples help or hinder patient safety efforts.

Physician leaders also have a critical stake in this matter. As I work on physician leadership development and physician engagement with many clients, I see how attention to patient safety and quality can gain the attention of physicians. Nonclinical leaders who pay heed to patient safety gain great credibility with their clinical colleagues. As I recruit physician leaders as well, I am often comforted to know that even those physicians who have left clinical practice still have patients in mind as they lead their healthcare organizations. So many physicians tell me in interviews that one of the primary reasons they enter the leadership ranks is the ability to affect patient safety, patient quality, and patient care at a broader level.

I applaud this book and its content. It contains many interesting bits of advice and counsel, numerous specific examples and real-world insights. It is well presented, well written, and compelling, and it will certainly be useful to all healthcare leaders. It is also a book you can pick up and pick a chapter and read. Each chapter is self-contained and has much for readers to glean.

Carson F. Dye, FACHE
President and CEO, Exceptional Leadership LLC

Preface

MEDICAL ERRORS CAUSE more than 200,000 deaths each year and are now the third leading cause of death in the United States (Cha 2016). Medical errors are mistakes that we make—and they are preventable.

You may know all of this, and you may even be numb from hearing it so often. You are not alone if you feel this way.

You might also be thinking that

- errors don't happen in my hospital;
- the medical error issue is so complicated, we can't do anything about it;
- we can't fix it; or
- the problem feels overwhelming.

But what if it isn't? What if it is changeable? Would it be worth your time?

If you are among the believers that preventable errors do not occur in your hospital or health system, think back. You have heard about some of these mistakes in your own hospital. You may have witnessed one as it unfolded. But picture this:

> It's 1980, and I [J.B.] am a medical student. I'm taking the board certification examination, and in walks the dean of the school. She pulls me into the hallway and tells me my grandfather has been in an accident. When I arrived

> at the emergency room, I saw my professor taking care of my grandfather. He was one of the professors I most respected.
>
> When I was growing up, Grandpa lived two doors down from me and my family. He built the house we lived in. My dad worked for the government and was gone a lot. So, Grandpa was a father to me.
>
> Day 1 went well; day 2 and day 3 went well. Then on day 4, my professor said we had a problem the previous night. He said, "Your grandpa's kidneys have failed; your grandpa won't be coming home."
>
> The nurse had given him a new nitroglycerin patch and failed to remove the old one. Grandpa died three days later.

Healthcare delivery does not have to be this way. Devastatingly poor outcomes do not need to happen. How do we know? Because making hospitals safe is what Susan and I do.

Many observers, practitioners, and staff are convinced that eliminating preventable harm is not achievable. Others believe errors are just a natural hazard of medical practice. If you feel we cannot fix these problems, consider this: At a children's hospital, our team helped the organization's staff cut serious errors by 90 percent. No more children have died because of medical errors at that hospital. At another hospital, as a result of the methods, tools, techniques, and processes we implemented, the organization has not experienced a serious error in more than 835 days, as of this writing. And reports of similar successes are coming in from hospitals all over the United States.

Imagine your hospital with zero errors. In addition to lives saved, that means no more disclosures, no more family conferences in which you must tell loved ones, "We caused the death of your family member."

Like Susan and me, you went into healthcare because you deeply care about people. Healthcare is a noble profession, in which people trust us with their lives at a time that they are the most vulnerable—at a time that they need our help.

We cannot fail them.

Together, we will make sure we deliver the safest care possible. Join us, and we will take the errors out of patient care.

YOUR *SAFETY PLAYBOOK* FOR DELIVERING ERROR-FREE CARE

Susan and I wrote this book as a practical guide for implementing a high-reliability safety program in a real-life healthcare environment. Our goal is to equip you with the know-how, tools, tactics, and strategies to build a safety program that eradicates preventable medical errors.

The Safety Playbook helps you create safe care environments for your patients, their families, *your* family, and your community. This book describes a comprehensive approach for healthcare organizations that brings them to the top of the nation's rating lists. It helps you do what most organizations have been unable to do on their own: Deliver error-free care at an affordable cost—true healthcare value.

The book is divided into seven parts as follows.

Part I: The US Patient Safety Crisis

This section establishes a common understanding of current death rates and provides an overview of several effective solutions. Ways to ignite a cultural shift in healthcare are introduced, and common beliefs are challenged. For instance, part I provides compelling evidence that (1) medical errors can be eliminated and (2) traditional improvement techniques may not be effective solutions.

Part II: Executing a Shift to Full Transparency

Transparency about performance, errors, and the causes of errors is central to a successful safety and high-reliability program. This section discusses the philosophy of full transparency, including benefits to organizations and their stakeholders. We also introduce several metrics and dashboards that can be immediately implemented in organizations.

Part III: Positions and New Roles

Effective safety programs depend on significant changes in the way physicians and staff perform their daily duties, and some will adopt completely different roles. For instance, some clinical staff may become safety coaches or trainers in the organization, developing skills that help the organization lower costs and ease the deployment of a safety culture transformation. This section covers many of the roles and key positions needed for success.

Part IV: Tools

Many safety tools that are used in other industries can be successfully adopted by healthcare. Tools and practices from airlines, nuclear power plants, and aircraft carriers are reviewed. Although some of these tools see widespread use in healthcare, even more do not. For each tool, evidence of its effectiveness is provided using case studies from a number of industries, including healthcare.

Part V: Communication

An entire section of the book is devoted to communication because miscommunication is the most common cause of medical errors.

Numerous effective communication strategies are highlighted, and case studies are provided to show how to implement these communication strategies, with supporting data demonstrating their effectiveness.

Part VI: Guidelines

Guidelines are effective tools used throughout healthcare, and several can support a culture of safety. Topics such as red rules, just culture, and the bottle-to-throttle rule are reviewed, among others.

Part VII: Bringing It All Together

This section provides a sample project plan along with a special section for chief financial officers that addresses resource needs for effective programs. A list of useful resources is provided at the end of the book.

Acknowledgments

The opening portion of the preface is adapted from the introduction of a popular keynote speech by John Byrnes. We extend special thanks to Amy Port for helping turn a rough draft into a polished, professional speech.

PART I

THE US PATIENT SAFETY CRISIS

CHAPTER 1

A Call to Action: The US Patient Safety Crisis[1]

A SAFETY CRISIS is brewing in healthcare. Medical errors currently rank third among causes of death in the United States (exhibit 1.1), with 210,000 to 440,000 US residents dying each year from preventable hospital medical errors (Cha 2016; James 2013).

Exhibit 1.1: Leading Causes of Death in the United States

1. Cardiovascular disease	611,105
2. Cancer	584,881
3. Medical errors	220,000–440,000
4. Chronic lower respiratory disease	149,205
5. Accidents	130,557
6. Stroke	128,978
7. Alzheimer's disease	84,767
8. Diabetes	75,578
9. Influenza and pneumonia	56,979
10. Kidney disease	47,112
11. Suicide	41,149

Source: CDC (2017b).

Healthcare safety programs have evolved over the past 20 years, and many organizations have made progress. However, many more struggle to provide consistently safe, high-quality care. In its 2016 nationwide safety survey of hospitals, the Leapfrog Group found that 40 percent received a C, a D, or an F rating in hospital safety.

CURRENT STATE OF SAFETY

As part of an ongoing effort to determine the reasons so many hospitals receive poor safety grades, one of the authors (J.B.) conducted a workshop with about 30 finance leaders from hospitals across the United States. The specific aims were to (1) explore the organizational factors that lead to lapses in safety or occurrences of sentinel events and (2) find out where patient safety ranks as a priority for healthcare finance executives.

To establish context for the discussion, the following information was shared with the group:

- Preventable adverse events account for "roughly one-sixth of all deaths that occur in the U.S. each year" (James 2013).
- More than 1,000 people die every day from preventable accidents in hospitals (McCann 2014).
- Errors of omission and commission, complications, readmissions, and avoidable mortality cost the US economy billions of dollars each year (Zajac 2009).
- On average, a hospitalized patient in the United States experiences at least one medication-related error—the most common type of error—each day (IOM 2007).
- In 2011, an estimated 722,000 hospital-acquired infections (HAIs) occurred in US acute care hospitals, and approximately 75,000 patients with HAIs died during their hospitalizations (CDC 2016).

- Among all US acute care hospitals, a report based on 2014 data found a 17 percent decrease in surgical site infections (SSIs). However, SSIs and pneumonia are still the most frequently occurring HAIs, afflicting an estimated 157,500 patients per year (CDC 2016).

Key Takeaways

As discussion ensued at the workshop, several key issues became apparent. More than a handful of leaders were unaware that preventable adverse events in hospitals rank so highly among the leading causes of death in the United States. Although all the participants knew the ranking was higher than acceptable, their lack of awareness about exactly how high signaled a great need to educate healthcare organizations—from the board to the front line—about this crisis.

Furthermore, many of the finance leaders in attendance did not realize they already had most of the data needed to study their organization's own errors, complications, readmissions, and mortality rates. Much of this information can be found in the incident-reporting and finance or cost accounting systems of every hospital.

Most acknowledged that their physician and nursing leaders likely lacked adequate training in safety science, the characteristics of high-reliability organizations (HROs), and process design to feel comfortable tackling the reduction of patient harm. Safety science and HRO design were not part of the clinical and educational curriculum when most individuals currently serving in leadership positions were trained in their clinical discipline.

When asked how much money the finance leaders were willing to invest to remove medical errors as a leading cause of death nationwide, several said, "Whatever it takes." But some were noncommittal when pressed to name an investment level they would support.

About half the leaders in attendance felt patient safety was a priority in their organization. But only a few described it as the top priority. By the end of the workshop, most felt it should be the number one priority, given the facts they now had in hand.

Finally, when asked, "Is safety discussed at every executive leadership meeting?" most said "no." While the workshop survey was not scientific, the discussion seemed to align with the findings of most reported hospital safety scores.

SOLUTIONS WITHIN REACH

Many organizations still have significant work ahead to solve the safety crisis, requiring a focused effort, committed executive teams, and the willingness to invest the necessary resources.

That said, the resource investment is less significant than many executives expect. For instance, in the authors' experience, among average-sized community hospitals, the net addition of three or fewer full-time-equivalent (FTE) staff members can help achieve gains in safety. However, although only a few new staff may be needed, they—along with the entire workforce—need to be trained in safety science and operational process redesign.

The healthcare workforce is missing an entire body of knowledge in safety science and process redesign, and gaining that knowledge is the most obvious solution to the healthcare safety crisis. Once organizations gain the necessary skills to operate safely and efficiently, the healthcare system will have solved a huge part of the problem.

In addition to strong, effective senior leadership and unwavering commitment, then, the effort requires a cultural transformation (the topic of chapter 2) to an HRO-level status and investment in organization-wide training.

To solve this crisis, each individual in the organization is responsible for accomplishing and sustaining zero patient harm. We know the US healthcare system can do better. Together we can make healthcare much safer for everyone.

NOTE

1. Portions of this chapter have been adapted from Byrnes (2015b) and Byrnes (2015c).

CHAPTER 2

Transformation to a Safety Culture

Culture has been defined as the arts and other manifestations of human intellectual achievement regarded collectively. Another definition is the sum of ways by which a particular population lives that has been built over time and transmitted from one generation to the next.

The notion of patient safety culture was introduced following publication of the Institute of Medicine's (IOM) landmark report, *To Err Is Human: Building a Safer Health System*, in 2000. This report encourages healthcare systems to "create an environment in which safety is a top priority driven by leadership." It describes a safety culture as one that focuses on preventing, detecting, and minimizing hazards and error without attaching blame to individuals.

Thus, understanding patient safety culture and how to achieve it is a relatively new area of study. Research conducted thus far generally supports a number of components in the process of building a culture of safety, but as with any sociological element, culture can be highly correlated with the people who are a part of it (Sammer and James 2011), meaning the people involved are seen as the cultural "bundle" in healthcare, just as clinical practices have process bundles.

KEYS TO SAFETY CULTURE TRANSFORMATION

Leadership is a key aspect of success in improving safety culture outcomes. Senior leaders must collectively commit to integrating high-reliability tactics into their own daily work. Such tactics include rounding to influence, whereby leaders are visible and interact with operations and frontline staff at the microsystem level on a regular basis. In an HRO, structures are set in place to inform senior leaders of any safety risks and to update them on safety metrics and improvement efforts. Deference to the expertise of individuals—staff and leaders alike—is another requirement for an organization to achieve improvements in safety, and it is cultivated through regular, open discussions with all levels of leadership and staff. Such ongoing vigilance is the only way to sustain initial gains that take place. Leadership is also responsible for engaging the physician community and providing education, resources, and opportunities to be involved with safety culture improvements. More leadership tools and tactics are discussed in chapter 9.

A balanced and "right" culture for staff and physicians is an important factor as well (Marx 2017). Often referred to as a just culture, such an environment allows the organization to differentiate between individual and system failures, helping improve transparency and error reporting in conjuction with individual performance management. Healthcare has traditionally been a punitive environment, but punishing staff for errors prevents individuals from reporting concerns and mistakes, which then remain cloaked in secrecy. As the organization continues to encourage nonpunitive reporting, its leaders must keep in mind that some individuals may not be in the right role or the right department, as they have developed unsafe practices that put patients and the organization at risk. The concept of just culture is explained at length in chapter 31.

Communication is another key to building a reliable, safe culture. Structuring communication through assertion techniques, which allow staff to raise concerns in the face of a traditional hierarchy;

adopting tools such as patient handoff checklists and SBAR, or situation–background–assessment–recommendation; and conducting briefings, read-backs, and repeat-backs have proven to be effective techniques as demonstrated by a number of studies in the literature (Boyd et al. 2014; Pagano 2016). In addition to effective clinical communications, targeted dialogue must occur between the leaders and the physicians and staff. Communication modalities for safety culture processes include 5:1 positive feedback strategies, whereby leaders are encouraged to provide five positive pieces of feedback for every one negative portion of feedback; follow-up on event reporting; safety storytelling; and safety alerts.

Patient-centric cultures use their efforts in improving patient safety as a baseline for positive patient experiences. Organizations that have a strong record of providing an outstanding patient experience can build a reliable safety culture more easily than can hospitals and health systems that have demonstrated poor or uneven patient safety. One way to solidify a safety culture is to have patients and families participate in the culture improvements; this approach improves the level of acceptance of these improvements by leaders, staff, and physicians. Patients and families can share valuable information about their care and the care of their loved ones. Including them in rounds and care conferences ultimately decreases the chances that patients experience an error.

In 2001, 18-month-old Josie King died of dehydration and a wrongly administered narcotic at Johns Hopkins Hospital. Her mother, Sorrel, offered invaluable input into the development of a patient- and family-centered approach to rapid response (Ayd 2004). The rapid response approach involves identifying a small group of people, such as the unit charge nurse, hospital supervisor, and hospitalist or division fellow physician, to respond to a patient or family member who feels he or she is not being heard regarding a concern.

Another approach to improving safety culture is the sharing of safety stories. Telling stories from across the healthcare system can powerfully engage staff and physicians because the stories help dispel the myth that "this could not happen here." Staff need to know that errors and events do happen in their organization, and storytelling not only reinforces that recognition but also offers lessons on how other staff worked to prevent them from recurring. Staff and physicians are compassionate professionals who want to take exceptional care of patients. A compassionate culture is one in which, at the very least, a patient is not harmed (Sammer and James 2011).

Transparency is crucial for a safety culture to develop. To build a culture characterized by transparency, metrics related to safety need to be gathered and made available to both leaders and staff, accompanied by easy-to-understand education about their meaning. The education required to establish and sustain transparency in turn suggests that the hospital or health system must become a learning organization. One often-overlooked aspect of organizational learning is the need to continually reinforce, through training and other events, the practice of asking *why*, rather than *who*, when events and errors occur. The organization needs to mobilize resources toward the prevention of recurrence and have mechanisms in place to discuss the events with all levels of the organization.

Transparency also must exist between the clinicians and the patients and families. Building an environment of transparency is not easy to accomplish. An essential starting point is to understand where the organization is in terms of current transparency levels. Leaders need to understand the importance of—and embrace—broad-based transparency and then work throughout the organization to continually improve transparency.

Multidisciplinary, multigenerational teamwork supports patient safety culture. Embedded in this notion is, again, deference to expertise: the integration of frontline staff into decision-making processes. Research has shown that encouraging the engagement of all disciplines when conducting bedside physician rounding improves outcomes and builds trust among the team members (Mittal et al. 2010). Improved teamwork in turn can flatten the healthcare hierarchy that exists and encourage a questioning attitude in the team. Attaining this level of psychological safety is also imperative to building resilience when errors and events do occur.

Related to deference to expertise is the prerequisite of establishing a culture of respect. Doing so is a complex endeavor, requiring leaders to motivate and engage team members and physicians at all levels to address issues of intimidation, physical safety, and environmental safety. Each person working in the organization needs to feel he or she is an appreciated part of the team.

In the next chapter, we look at successful case studies throughout the United States in building a culture of safety. In general, each of these organizations took a stepwise approach to improving their culture of safety toward becoming an HRO. Some of the approaches they adopted on this journey are an assessment of their current state, the development of high-capacity leadership functions and methods, education regarding safety science and high-reliability tools and methods, the encouragement of incident reporting, a build-up of cause analysis capabilities, the development of a safety metrics dashboard, and the use of in situ simulation. Readers will learn more about each of these methods and tools as we move down the high-reliability path throughout the book.

CHAPTER 3

Proof That This Formula Works: Results from Around the United States

THE IMPLEMENTATION OF safety programs and high-reliability efforts are showing incredible results. In the authors' experience, seeing serious safety event rates (SSERs) plummet by 25, 40, and even 90 percent in well-executed programs is not uncommon. Furthermore, the authors note that the benefits of such programs extend beyond decreased SSERs as organizations experience improvements in other patient safety and quality indicators.

Since 2012, Children's Hospitals' Solutions for Patient Safety (2017), a national effort to eliminate serious patient harm at children's hospitals, has saved 6,944 children from serious harm and reports a consistent upward trend in harm prevented every month, according to data as of September 2016.

Following are just a few of the organizations demonstrating the efficacy of the patient safety concept:

- Helen DeVos Children's Hospital (HDVCH), part of Spectrum Health, Grand Rapids, Michigan, has seen a 68 percent decrease in serious safety events (SSEs) in two years and a 90 percent decrease in SSERs at the four-year mark (Peterson, Teman, and Connors 2012).

- Children's National Medical Center, Washington, D.C., has experienced a 70 percent reduction in serious harm events (Hilliard et al. 2012).
- Nationwide Children's Hospital, Columbus, Ohio, reduced serious harm incidents by 83 percent (Brilli et al. 2013).
- VCU Medical Center, part of VCU Health, affiliated with Virginia Commonwealth University, Richmond, reduced its incidence of serious harm by 50 percent (Putre 2014).
- Sentara Healthcare, based in Suffolk, Virginia, has seen an 80 percent reduction in serious harm events overall, with a 50 percent reduction in harm events in 18 months (Putre 2014).

Next, we take a closer look at two of these high-performing sites: Nationwide Children's Hospital and Helen DeVos Children's Hospital.

CASE STUDY: NATIONWIDE CHILDREN'S HOSPITAL[1]

Nationwide Children's Hospital is a 610-bed pediatric hospital in Columbus, Ohio, with more than 1,280 medical staff members and over 10,000 total employees. In recent years, the hospital has been ranked as one of America's Best Children's Hospitals by *US News & World Report*. It is the pediatric teaching hospital for The Ohio State University College of Medicine (Nationwide Children's Hospital 2017a).

Beginning in 2008, Nationwide Children's set a goal to eliminate all preventable harm by 2013 by using a two-pronged approach: (1) effecting a safety culture transformation to become an HRO and (2) significantly expanding its quality and safety resources.

The Beginning

Nationwide Children's established a six-step process toward eliminating patient harm.

Step 1. Safety data were presented to the quality committee of the hospital's board of directors. This action included a call from the board to hospital management to drive "preventable harm to zero" and created a sense of urgency.

Step 2. Past SSEs were analyzed for common causes, and a variety of error prevention tools were developed to address the common causes found in their analysis.

Step 3. A training course in error prevention was developed, and 8,000 staff (clinical and nonclinical) and physicians participated. Additional training was provided to approximately 600 leaders. They received safety training on leadership methods and techniques to reinforce the HRO concepts taught during the more basic training.

Step 4. The root cause analysis process was improved, and system failures that were identified triggered corrective action plans.

Step 5. A safety coach program was launched for frontline staff so they could coach their peers on the effective use of the error prevention techniques and safety tools.

Step 6. Internal and external transparency, supported by executive leadership and the board of directors, was significantly increased. Safety data were posted to the Nationwide Children's intranet, and in November 2011, the hospital posted its SSER on its external website (exhibit 3.1).

Quality Infrastructure, Tools, and Teams

Nationwide Children's made a substantial investment in staffing and infrastructure to support its safety program. The budget was increased from $690,000 in 2007 to $3.3 million by 2012. The

Exhibit 3.1: Serious Safety Event Rate, Nationwide Children's Hospital, July 2009–October 2016

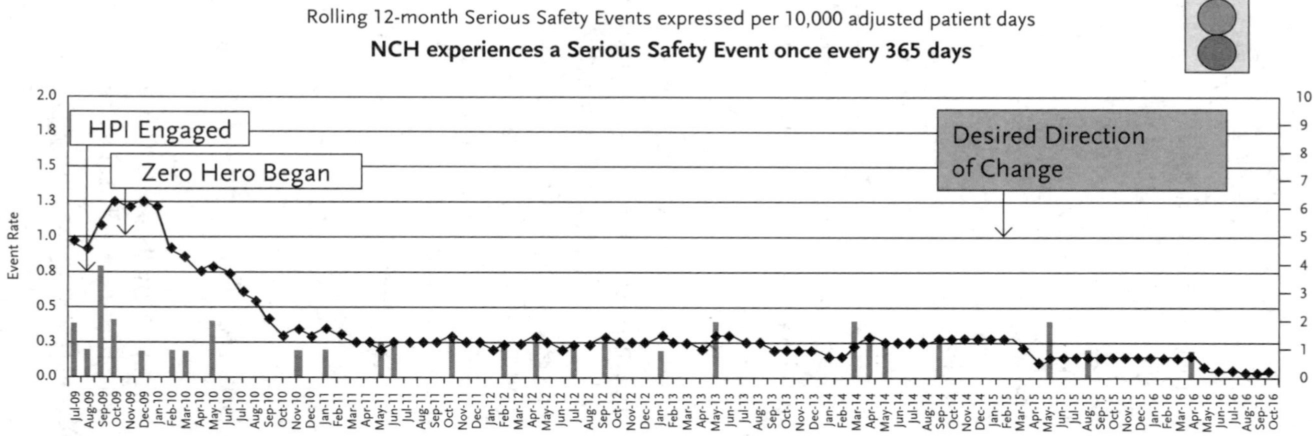

Source: Reprinted with permission from Nationwide Children's Hospital (2017b).
Note: Zero hour marks the beginning of the SSER rate-tracking initiative. HPI = Healthcare Performance Improvement; NCH = Nationwide Children's Hospital.

number of personnel in the quality improvement (QI) department was increased from 8 in 2007 to 33 by 2012, and many QI analysts were hired from industries outside of healthcare.

Harm detection was augmented with trigger tools, an upgraded event-reporting system, pharmacy interventions, and the analysis of complaints and grievances. Hospital leadership found that the greatest source of harm reports came from the event-reporting system, and the number of reports increased by 35 percent between 2009 and 2012.

Multidisciplinary teams were formed to target harm events, which included the most common events at Nationwide Children's Hospital (2017b): pressure ulcers (PUs), adverse drug events (ADEs), and hospital-acquired infections (HAIs).

The PU team introduced the following measures for tackling skin ulcers:

- Unit-based skin teams were created consisting of unit nursing staff, educators, wound ostomy care nurses, and a QI analyst.
- A PU prevention bundle was developed, and bundle compliance was measured and posted on nursing units. Units with low bundle compliance produced written action plans on how to improve.

The ADE reduction team focused on medication utilization (i.e., administration, prescribing, dispensing, and monitoring) in the intensive care units (ICUs) and then hospitalwide. Interventions included the following:

- Development of an ADE prevention bundle
- Implementation of a wireless communication system to quickly locate a second nurse to verify critical medicine administration
- Establishment of post-ADE huddles

- Use of medication pumps with dose-range checking and bar coding
- Placement of medication safety champions on each unit to reinforce medication-related safety behaviors

Nationwide Children's chartered a multidisciplinary team for each type of HAI. In general, each team created prevention bundles, measured compliance, and instituted formal debriefings each time an infection occurred. Central line–associated bloodstream infection (CLABSI) prevention included hospitalwide use of the Children's Hospital Association insertion and maintenance bundle. Catheter-associated urinary tract infection (CAUTI) prevention efforts targeted reductions in catheter days, standardized insertion techniques, and measured compliance with insertion and maintenance care bundles.

Results at Nationwide Children's Hospital

Serious Safety Events

A significant decrease in SSEs occurred as the program matured. As reported in the December 2013 issue of the *Journal of Pediatrics* (Brilli et al. 2013), "the number of SSEs per quarter decreased by 85.1%, from 6.7 to 1.0 (P < .001). . . . [A]n estimated 63 SSEs were prevented over the past 11 quarters. The SSER decreased from a peak of 1.15 in November 2009 to 0.19 by March 2011, an 83.3% decrease (P < .001)" (see exhibit 3.2). The article notes, "This rate reduction was sustained for 22 consecutive months, through January 2013." As shown earlier in exhibit 3.1, this performance has been maintained through 2016.

Pressure Ulcers

As expected, the rate of PUs increased in 2011 as a result of improved detection. The rate then decreased from a mean of 0.55 PUs per 1,000 patient days to a mean of 0.31 in 2012 ($p < .009$). Nationwide

Children's notes that the decrease coincided with an increase in inpatient PU prevention bundle compliance, from 55 percent in January 2011 to 80 percent in December 2012.

Adverse Drug Events

As with PUs, the rate of ADEs increased initially as the result of improved detection; it then began to decrease significantly in February 2011, with the mean number of ADEs per 1,000 dispensed doses decreasing from 0.17 to 0.09 ($p < .001$). Furthermore, ADE bundle compliance has reached, sustained, and regularly exceeds 90 percent compliance since October 2010.

Hospital-Acquired Infections

Although not statistically significant, Nationwide Children's found that annually, HAIs decreased from 76 in 2009 to 50 in 2012. Among the hospital's accomplishments in this area, the pediatric ICU had

Exhibit 3.2: SSER and Number of SSEs, 2009–2013

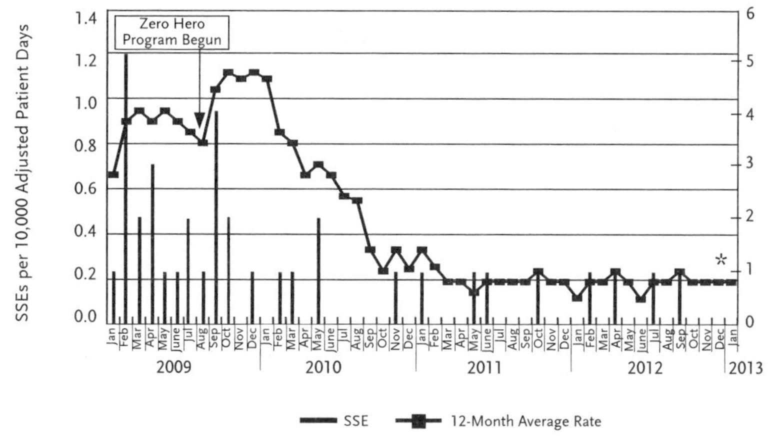

Source: Brilli et al. (2013).
Note: SSE = serious safety event; SSER = serious safety event rate. Zero hour marks the start of the SSE initiative. Bars represent number of monthly SSEs; line represents 12-month rolling average of SSEs per 10,000 adjusted patient days.
$^{*}p < .001$.

achieved more than 800 consecutive days without a CLABSI as of the time of this writing, and hospitalwide CLABSI, CAUTI, and surgical site infection rates all decreased, albeit not to a statistically significant point, while hospital ventilator-acquired pneumonia (VAP) rates decreased from 0.04 per 1,000 ventilator days in 2009 to 0.0 in 2012 ($p < .01$).

As demonstrated by these and other outcomes, Nationwide Children's HRO program is a success.

CASE STUDY: HELEN DEVOS CHILDREN'S HOSPITAL[2]

Helen DeVos Children's Hospital (HDVCH), a 200-bed tertiary-care hospital in Grand Rapids, Michigan, began its safety culture transformation in fall 2007, when hospital president Robert Connors, MD, charged the entire hospital staff, including physicians, with making HDVCH the safest pediatric hospital in the nation.

Safety Culture Transformation Steps

As with Nationwide Children's and most other successfully transformative healthcare organizations, HDVCH established a stepwise approach to hardwire its safety program and culture.

Step 1: Launch a Safety Culture Model

Senior leaders at HDVCH introduced a safety culture model to launch its safety program. The model was built on the following components:

- Safety education and training for all staff, including physicians
- Training in root cause analysis and failure mode and effects analysis of safety events and behaviors for all staff

- Safety toolkit development for staff and management
- Full integration of and collaboration among risk management and clinical staff
- Consistent coding and classification of SSEs
- Adoption of a set of safety metrics
- Fostering of transparency of data and safety event details

Step 2: Establish and Track a Serious Safety Event Rate Metric

This stage of the process included the following elements:

- Full disclosure of all sentinel events at HDVCH between 2005 and 2007
- Extensive review of the events using common cause analysis and failure mode taxonomies
- Documentation and scoring of system- and human-based errors
- Creation of a baseline SSE rate
- Tracking of near-miss events, or deviations from the standard of care that did not reach the patient, and precursor events, or incidents from which deviations from the standard of care reached the patient but did not cause serious harm

Step 3: Train All Staff in Safety Behaviors

More than 4,000 clinical and administrative staff participated in a two-hour workshop on basic safety behaviors and received the aforementioned safety toolkits. The tools were selected according to the most common issues discovered in the common cause analysis in step 2. These tools include peer and self-checking, clarification and questioning for clear communication, attention to detail, and review.

Training was reinforced through practice, regular feedback by unit-based safety coaches, blog posts about safety, posted safety updates, "good catch" reports, and rounding by the safety coaches.

Unit-based safety coaches developed expertise through additional training and practice in essential safety behaviors. They then coached and mentored frontline staff in their respective units.

Specialized training in cause analysis was offered to select individuals who could participate in event analysis, including unit-based nurses, physicians, infection control staff, respiratory therapists, and other area staff.

Step 4: Reinforce Accountability

Events that resulted in serious patient harm required immediate oversight by the risk management department and patient safety specialists. Less serious events were followed by unit-level cause analysis.

The serious patient harm cases were assigned to an executive, who developed an action plan for achievements at 30-, 60-, and 90-day increments. The executive was supported by a team including risk management staff and patient safety specialists.

Step 5: Institutionalize Transparency

Organization-wide transparency was quickly accomplished by incorporating the discussion of safety metrics into regular meetings of the hospital's board of directors; executive leaders; department chiefs; nursing and quality improvement leaders; and all clinical and nonclinical staff, risk management personnel, and legal counsel.

In addition to the SSER, metrics that were adopted included days since the last SSE, number of near-miss and precursor events, and SSE-to–precursor event ratio.

Step 6: Prioritize Safety Issues

A top-10 list of the most immediate and highest priority issues was created. Each issue on the list was assigned an owner, and the owner reported on progress every week for the next 18 months at an executive safety committee (exhibit 3.3) chaired by HDVCH's chief operating officer. This list also helped promote an enhanced level of accountability.

Exhibit 3.3: Top-10 List of Safety Priorities at Helen DeVos Children's Hospital

1. Medication errors
2. Ventilator-associated pneumonia
3. Rates of asthma core measurement requirements met
4. Patient satisfaction rates
5. Employee satisfaction rates
6. Hand hygiene compliance
7. Quality of low-volume and high-risk specialty care
8. Retinopathy of prematurity in the neonatal ICU
9. Smart pump use
10. Catheter-associated blood stream infections in the pediatric ICU

Source: Reprinted with permission from Peterson, Teman, and Connors (2012).
Note: ICU = intensive care unit.

Results

Common Cause Analysis

The leading system-based causes for failures included culture (e.g., not voicing a concern because of intimidation), at 54 percent; poorly developed or nonexistent processes, at 23 percent; and faulty or absent policies and protocols, at 12 percent. Common human error causes included failure to employ critical thinking (33 percent), normalized deviance (21 percent), and poor communication and failure to attend to detail (17 percent each).

Serious Safety Event Rate

The baseline SSER was 0.81 per 10,000 patient days at the end of the training phase. By December 2009, the rate had decreased by 68 percent to a low of 0.26 per 10,000 (exhibit 3.4).

Exhibit 3.4: Rolling 12-Month Rate per 10,000 Adjusted Patient Days, February 2007–November 2010

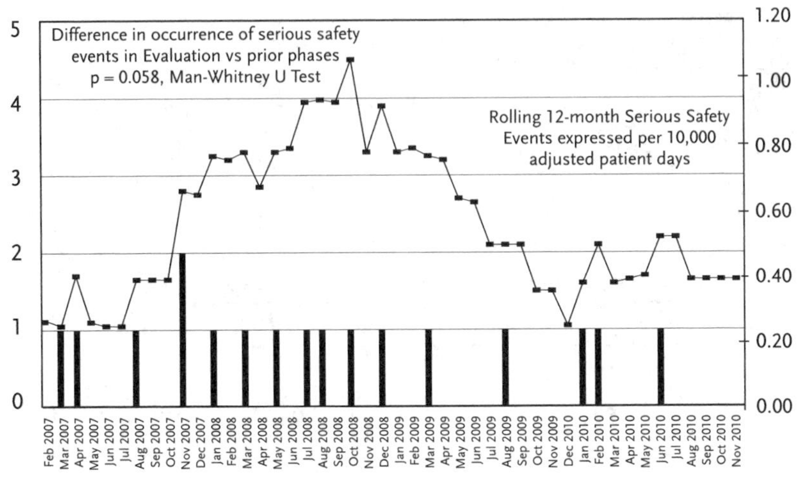

Source: Reprinted with permission from Peterson, Teman, and Connors (2012).

Ventilator-Acquired Pneumonia

In the HDVCH pediatric critical care unit, baseline compliance with the VAP bundle was 2 percent. Within six months of the launch of the safety program, the bundle compliance rate was 96 percent, and no VAP events occurred in that time frame (exhibit 3.5). This outcome was likely due to this issue's placement on the top-10 list. In addition, only one VAP case was experienced in the subsequent 12 months, yielding a rate of 0.53 per 1,000 ventilator days at the end of 2009.

Hand Washing and Hospital-Acquired Infections

Handwashing compliance was also placed on the top-10 list when rates were measured at 56 percent. Again, within six months of the safety interventions, the rate rose above 95 percent and remains in the mid- to upper 90 percent range (exhibit 3.6). Concurrently, HAIs dropped by 50 percent.

Exhibit 3.5: Ventilator-Associated Pneumonia Bundle Compliance Rate, PICU, January 2008–December 2009

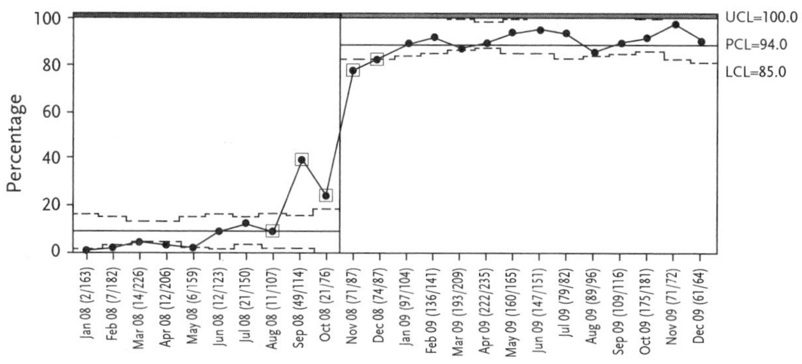

Source: Reprinted with permission from Peterson, Teman, and Connors (2012).
Note: Rate calculated by the number of patients whose cases were compliant with the bundle divided by the total number of patients on a ventilator. The upper control limit (UCL) and lower control limit (LCL) indicate 3 standard deviations from the mean or process center line (PCL); PICU = pediatric intensive care unit.

Exhibit 3.6: Hand-Hygiene Compliance Rate, PICU, January 2008–December 2009

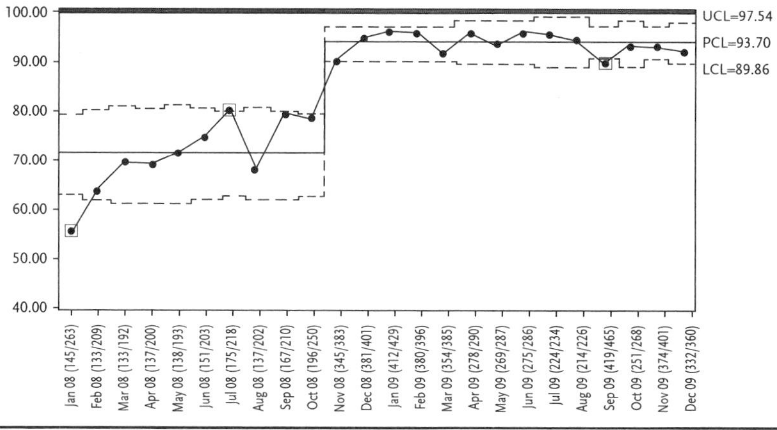

Source: Reprinted with permission from Peterson, Teman, and Connors (2012).
Note: Rate calculated by the number of hospital staff who performed appropriate hand hygiene divided by the total number of hospital staff observed. The upper control limit (UCL) and lower control limit (LCL) indicate 3 standard deviations from the mean or process center line (PCL); lower warning limit indicates 2 standard deviations. PICU = pediatric intensive care unit.

NOTES

1. Information regarding the Nationwide Children's case study was obtained from Brilli et al. (2013) unless otherwise noted.
2. Information regarding the HDVCH case study was obtained from Peterson, Teman, and Connors (2012) unless otherwise noted.

CHAPTER 4

The Need for High Reliability

A HIGH-RELIABILITY ORGANIZATION is one that has succeeded in avoiding catastrophes in an environment where accidents are expected due to risk factors related to, and the complexity of, operational processes. Karl Weick and Kathleen Sutcliffe (2015), authors of *Managing the Unexpected*, state that in addition to having a unique structure, HROs also adopt different thought processes and act differently from other organizations. HROs use mindful organizing for the unexpected as well as the expected. Simply put, HROs are hazardous environments where the consequences of errors are high but the occurrence of error is extremely low (Loeb and Chassin 2013).

Historically, the airline and nuclear power industries and naval nuclear submarine builders have been known as HROs. In early 2013, the Aviation Safety Network (ASN) reported that 2012 was "the safest year for air travel since 1945." Worldwide, 23 crashes occurred in that year—or one fatal crash per every 2.5 million flights—resulting in 475 air fatalities and 36 ground fatalities. These numbers represent a tremendous improvement over the previous ten-year average of 34 fatal crashes and 773 deaths (ASN 2013).

The airline industry has made such significant strides in safety and reliability in part by adhering to the International Aviation Safety Assessment program, which is composed of the following eight elements (FAA 2016):

CE-1. Primary aviation legislation
CE-2. Specific operating regulations
CE-3. State civil aviation system and safety oversight functions
CE-4. Technical personnel qualification and training
CE-5. Technical guidance, tools, and the provision of safety-critical information
CE-6. Licensing, certification, authorization, and approval obligations
CE-7. Surveillance obligations
CE-8. Resolution of safety concerns

In the nuclear power industry, safety is associated with, but addressed separately from, security. Safety programs focus on unintended conditions or events leading to radiological releases from authorized activities, meaning safety relates mainly to internal problems or hazards. In a complementary fashion, security focuses on the intentional misuse of nuclear or other radioactive materials by nonstate (nongovernment) elements to cause harm. Security programs relate mainly to external threats to materials or facilities, and safeguards are concerned with restraining activities by nation-states that could lead to acquisition of nuclear weapons—materials and equipment in the hands of rogue governments.

Safety and security for naval nuclear-powered submarines mirror those activities undertaken in power plants, including prioritizing high levels of standardization, find-and-fix exercises, and teamwork.

What can healthcare learn from these organizations? Can some of their safety processes, tools, and tactics be implemented in hospitals and health systems? They can. To perform in the manner of HROs in other industries, healthcare organizations must have a solid understanding of the elements of high reliability set out by Weick and Sutcliffe (2015) and use that knowledge to apply the specific tools and training. The nuclear power and airline industries have these five elements in place, and healthcare can improve by building them into all its organizations.

The first three elements involve the anticipation of failure:

- *Preoccupation with failure.* To avoid failure, organizations must look for failure and be sensitive to its early signs.
- *Reluctance to simplify.* Rather than try to resolve issues by looking for superficial causes, leaders should plan to view safety lapses through a highly critical lens that brings to the surface the deeper solutions.
- *Sensitivity to operations.* Systems are not static and linear but rather dynamic and nonlinear. HROs are highly aware of what the next 24 hours will bring and where weaknesses exist in the system.

The last two elements detailed by Weick and Sutcliffe relate to the importance of having the ability to contain errors and failures. Containment involves the following traits:

- *Commitment to resilience.* The organization must maintain functioning during high-demand events. Resilience has three components:
  - Absorb strain and preserve function despite adversity.
  - Maintain the ability to return to service from serious events.
  - Learn and grow from previous events.
- *Deference to expertise.* Deference should cascade downward to frontline members of the organization. An example of deference to expertise is involving bedside nurses in improvement processes that relate to their clinical area of practice. Credibility, a necessary component of expertise, is the mutual recognition of skill levels and legitimacy. Deference also includes arming staff at the front line with the ability to identify concerns toward further containment of errors as well as addressing them.

Another view of high reliability, offered by Baker, Day, and Salas (2006), includes respectful interaction on the basis of trust, honesty, and self-respect. Respectful interaction is built over time; must be driven by leaders in the highest level of the organization; and is founded on a culture that is just, learning, flexible, and transparent. Furthermore, in our experience, members of the HRO feel they are supported in reporting incidents and events, lessons are learned from all events that are reported, and discussions regarding events are shared at all levels of the organization.

The Agency for Healthcare Research and Quality outlines the case example of Sentara Leigh Hospital in Norfolk, Virginia (Hines et al. 2008). Sentara Leigh coupled high-reliability concepts and innovations to improve patient safety outcomes. These included implementing no-interruption zones around its medication dispensing machines and improving communication within and between teams through check-in meetings, nurse huddles, and executive walk-arounds. Additional organizational results are broadly described in chapter 5.

As mentioned earlier, becoming an HRO involves a combination of structure and function. Loeb and Chassin (2013) describe the three high-level ingredients for integrating high-reliability principles into hospitals and healthcare organizations. First is the leadership's commitment to the ultimate goal of zero patient harm. Next is the incorporation of all the principles and practices of a safety culture throughout the organization. Third is the widespread adoption and deployment of the most effective process improvement tools and methods.

Leadership methods for hardwiring these elements include executive walk-arounds, a safety-first mentality, find-and-fix applications, strong cause analysis methods, an absence of hierarchy issues, a just culture, transparency in safety metrics, and investment in process improvements (Gamble 2013). Other organizational tools include "stop the line," visual management, peer accountability, structured communication, and teamwork methods. These leadership methods and tools are described throughout this book.

All HROs know that small things that go wrong are often early warning signals of deepening trouble and can provide insight into the health of the whole system. HROs also treat near misses and errors as information on the health of their system and try to learn from them. In general, healthcare systems have a long way to go to becoming HROs. Incremental change can bring organizations closer to the level of reliability experienced in the airline industry and nuclear power, and the first change must be for leaders to adopt a safety-first culture before the organization moves on to build the structures and functions that support improvement of outcomes on a reliable basis.

CHAPTER 5

Integrating Patient and Employee Safety

HEALTHCARE FACILITIES WHERE the staff have positive perceptions of workplace safety tend to have a positive assessment of patient safety culture (Mohr et al. 2015). This chapter examines employee safety metrics, types of employee safety, and similarities between employee safety and patient safety.

Traditionally, employee safety was referred to as occupational health, and hospitals and health systems employed occupational health nurses or operated whole departments dedicated to employee safety. Occupational health was initially concerned with injuries that occurred to staff while on the job. The definition has since expanded to include personal, physical, and emotional employee safety.

Personal safety includes issues such as workplace violence, pedestrian safety, and emergency preparedness. Hospitals and health systems mirror the cities in which they reside. If crime rates are high and substance abuse and mental health issues are prevalent in the community, the segment of the population that presents these issues in the hospital is likely high in number as well. The goal of personal safety initiatives is to reduce risk and anxiety for staff. Organizations should have in place visible security measures—security officers who round proactively and safe transportation to and from the campus buildings, for example—and should discuss personal safety with employees on an ongoing basis. Adequate funding and staffing is required for the assessment and monitoring of high-risk patients who require constant surveillance due to risk for violence to employees. A number of organizations have implemented staff safety and situational awareness training to enable staff to recognize and respond to escalating patient and visitor violence. Healthcare organizations are also required by state regulations and The Joint Commission, and other healthcare accrediting bodies, to have a plan for emergencies, including weather-related events, accidents, and community emergencies.

Physical safety closely resembles traditional occupational health. It covers such issues as needle sticks, strains and falls, workplace violence, and workplace ergonomics. The most recognized metric is "days away, restricted, or transferred" (DART), developed by the Occupational Safety and Health Administration (OSHA). It measures the number of injuries that result in days an employee is away from work, restrictions imposed on an employee's work activities, or transfers to another area that can accommodate an employee's work needs. The formula for DART is the number of injuries per calendar year multiplied by 200,000 then divided by the total number of hours worked in the same calendar year. Hospitals are becoming increasingly capable of capturing these data to understand the extent of employee physical safety issues.

Regarding emotional safety, research shows that 33 percent of nurses and 17 percent of physicians leave their profession after just one year of practice (Lucian Leape Institute 2015). Furthermore, 30 to 65 percent of healthcare workers report feeling burned out, with the highest rates experienced by physicians at the front line of care.

Many healthcare organizations have programs in place for the so-called second victim of medical errors—the healthcare worker, generally a clinician, who has experienced an error that leads to some degree of harm to the patient. Critical incident teams can be helpful in mitigating the stress of being a second victim. The teams are composed of specially trained staff from a variety of disciplines who respond quickly (within 48 hours) after an incident. They bring together the individuals who were caring for the patient at the time of the error and facilitate a discussion of what occurred and how the care providers are feeling. They offer a variety of resources, including employee assistance programs and follow-up for those who are interested or continue to struggle.

Failure to address second victims' emotional health and safety can lead to physical ailments, burnout, shame, and even depression and posttraumatic stress disorder. Caregivers may also experience moral distress. Moral distress can occur when caregivers feel they are unable to follow a correct course of action for a patient because of internal and external constraints. Hospitals need to have systems in place that allow staff and physicians to elevate these concerns and have them addressed in a timely fashion. Large organizations have ethics professionals and committees that assist in resolving these types of concerns.

The financial impact of employee injuries includes medical costs, lost and restricted days, replacement of employees, overtime, loss of expertise, and productivity delays. As with many initiatives, to adequately address employee safety, leaders must have knowledge and awareness of where the organization stands at the beginning—a baseline. The development of an initial DART score can be helpful in this effort. In addition, the Workplace Violence Staff Assessment Survey, developed by the American Society for Healthcare Risk Managers, can provide a second data set to start with.

The development of a team to design a comprehensive approach to employee safety can constitute the next level of measurement. This team can assist in building employee safety as a core value. It can also monitor the metrics gathered and report results to leadership.

Much like patient safety programs, comprehensive employee safety programs need to have elements of prevention, detection, and correction. The program may include but is not limited to rounding for employee safety; in-depth review of current technologies and processes; education on best practices; emergency preparedness; hospital security proactivity; office ergonomics assessments; American Nurses Association standards for safe patient handling and movement or mobility; management of slips, trips, and falls;

and cause analysis. Root cause analysis principles can be applied to staff incidents with the creation of action plans to assist in prevention of recurrence.

Other patient safety tools described in upcoming chapters apply to both employee and patient safety. As mentioned earlier, leadership rounds may feature discussions with staff about recent incidents or current concerns. Leaders can review feedback from patient safety and workplace safety surveys as a starting point for discussion. Education should be provided about awareness and recognition of high-risk situations, such as an unexpected patient death, protective services involvement with a pediatric patient, a patient with a history of aggression toward staff, or a patient with untreated mental illness or substance abuse. Peer checking and coaching may be applied in the use of safe patient-handling protocols. Staff may be educated in the culture of 200 percent accountability for employee safety—"I am 100 percent responsible for keeping myself safe and 100 percent accountable for keeping my teammates safe."

Organization-wide implementation of cause analysis programs for all employee injuries can prevent these types of injuries from recurring. Leaders and physicians should encourage the escalation of concerns by using safe phrase terminology—a red flag of sorts that everyone in the organization recognizes and uses when he or she has a concern that is not being addressed—or the implementation of a help chain.

In 2015, the National Patient Safety Foundation published a report titled *Shining a Light: Safer Healthcare Through Transparency*. The report is a compilation of recommendations to encourage support for all who work in healthcare. As stated in the publication, "workplace safety is inextricably linked to patient safety. Unless caregivers are given the protection, respect and support they need, they're more likely to make errors, fail to follow safe practices and not work well in teams." Using similar approaches to patient and employee safety allows for enhanced understanding among staff, enabling healthcare organizations to become highly reliable.

PART II

EXECUTING A SHIFT TO FULL TRANSPARENCY

CHAPTER 6

A Culture of Full Transparency and No-Fault Reporting

HIGHLY RELIABLE ORGANIZATIONS ask themselves, What strengths and weaknesses do we have in our system? What do we need to improve? What resources do we need to address these quality and competition concerns? To answer these questions on an ongoing basis, and to have confidence that they are getting the right information to do so, organizations need a high level of transparency. In a report from the Lucian Leape Institute (2015), transparency in a healthcare setting is described as an environment in which defects are made visible and learnings are shared freely and without inhibition.

What is the value of transparency in a high-reliability organization (HRO)? First, it is an ethically correct practice. Discussions about incidents, events, and issues must occur both within the organization and with patients and families. Patients deserve to know when an error has occurred and what the organization has done to address it.

Second, transparency can lead to and support improved patient outcomes. When issues are identified and subsequently resolved, chances are reduced that they will affect another patient.

Third, preventable-error rates are improved and costs are lowered through uncompromising transparency. Costs can come in the form of litigation and, increasingly, denials in reimbursement. Many insurers now decline to reimburse for hospital-acquired conditions and some readmissions because they are often a result of errors and misses in the system.

Fourth, transparency leads to improvement in patient satisfaction rates. Open, frank communication with patients is highly correlated with high patient satisfaction. Transparency coupled with the structured communication and teamwork approaches of HROs can improve the patient experience. When the organization has an expectation that clinicians will communicate thoroughly with each other, and has a structure in place for them to do so, patients benefit. Patients also appreciate open, honest, and complete information from their care team. When an organization values transparency, such openness can occur regularly.

Although the first value listed is the main reason most organizations work to build transparency, the others are key means for survival in modern healthcare. As organizations are increasingly reimbursed for patient outcomes in both clinical quality and patient experience, and considering reimbursement is withheld in certain error-driven patient events, those organizations that build a high level of transparency will not only survive but thrive.

Shekelle and colleagues (2013) describe several patient-centered safety and reliability strategies that can be implemented immediately. These strategies are supported in the research and current literature; examples offered in the "strongly encouraged" category include the use of checklists, bundles, and hand-hygiene practices. Under the "encouraged" category is "complementary methods for detecting adverse events or medical errors to monitor patient safety outcomes," in alignment with HROs' consistent treatment of near misses and errors as information about the health of the system and as teaching moments.

What tactics have been found to improve transparency in a healthcare organization? First, all stakeholders must have a common, solid understanding of the context of that organization. A better question, then, is, What works here? Institutions vary widely in their processes; often, the same can be said of institutional units, disciplines, and even like professionals. When assessing a current level of transparency, each segment needs to be honest about its starting point. Safety culture surveys can provide this type of feedback. If an organization already has a reporting system in place, the data it gathers can be helpful in defining a baseline metric to measure improvement in transparency. Important to realize is that while voluntary safety event systems do not provide a comprehensive accounting of all safety events, they serve an important function in building transparency. Chart review, trigger tool systems, huddles, and daily safety check-ins can all support the improvement of transparency.

A crucial aspect of instituting or improving a culture of transparency is recognizing why people in healthcare do not report safety events. A certain level of tolerance has been built into the healthcare environment toward medical errors. Clinicians have historically held a so-called known complication mentality toward nearly all errors and sentinel events, and any organization undergoing a shift to transparency must accept this mentality at the outset.

In addition, many healthcare cultures discourage open discussions of errors and learning from mistakes. In these cases, just culture—discussed in chapter 31—is absent. Healthcare has generally been known as a punitive rather than proactive environment in terms of addressing errors. To effect change toward adopting transparency, difficult communications and dedicated teamwork are required.

So, what specific steps can leaders take to improve transparency? First, they need to communicate why reporting errors is important. The message must be sent, repeated, and institutionalized that "We cannot fix what we don't know about" so members of the organization build a mentality of fixing the system.

Second, leaders need to treat employees justly and fairly. The first question HROs ask when a safety issue arises is, Why did this happen? rather than Who did it? One way to hardwire this mind-set is to discuss the event by referencing job titles rather than individuals' names (Gamble 2013). Just culture algorithms, examples of which are provided in chapter 31, can aid in the decision-making process for moving forward when an employee experiences an error.

Consistent application of an algorithm lessens the chance that employees will feel they are being treated differently than others when an event occurs.

Third, a robust lessons-learned program demonstrates to employees that leadership pays attention to error reporting and makes resources available to improve the system. Lessons-learned programs are discussed in detail in chapter 8.

Fourth, an essential component of a transparency program, especially in regard to error reporting, is a mechanism for reporting safety events that is easy for employees and physicians to use. A variety of electronic reporting systems are on the market and are generally far superior to a paper reporting system. That said, neither type of system supports transparency if it takes too much time to log a report or is too difficult to access.

Fifth, staff at all levels of the organization must be educated on what to report. Complications, system concerns, communication breakdowns, disruptive behavior, delays in care, environmental concerns, and area-specific issues are examples of the types of events that should be reported. Patient and family concerns also need a means to be captured, with specific follow-up and reporting specifications to the appropriate departments.

The Lucian Leape Institute (2015) report cited earlier also emphasizes the need for transparency beyond the reporting of events, presented in a sequence of levels or stages:

1. *Transparency among healthcare providers*—for example, case reviews for shared learning in the form of multidisciplinary conferences, as when a patient event has occurred.
2. *Transparency between clinicians and patients*—in the form of disclosure when an error has been experienced, whether or not a poor outcome resulted.
3. *Transparency of healthcare organizations with one another*—in the form of regional or national collaboratives. This level of transparency is increasingly occurring under the umbrella of patient safety organizations (PSOs).

4. *Transparency of both clinicians and organizations with the public*—for example, by providing easy access to patient quality and safety outcomes data.

The report also provides a summary of 33 recommendations for healthcare organizations to consider and implement.

Healthcare organizations that increase transparency in every area improve trust and ethical behavior; build a system by which to prioritize quality and safety interventions; and improve communications with patients and families, thereby improving the patient experience (Botwinick, Bisognano, and Haraden 2006). To start on the road to high reliability, building transparency needs to be among the first interventions an organization implements. A combination of cultural changes and visible metrics can lead the way.

CHAPTER 7

Safety Metrics

HIGH-RELIABILITY ORGANIZATIONS WORK to decrease errors as well as the degree of harm in their complex systems. In the ongoing effort to become highly reliable, exceptional organizations collect, analyze, and disseminate safety metrics to understand the extent to which they meet this overarching goal (Vogus and Sutcliffe 2007).

As yet, no standardized set of metrics for safety has been developed for organizations to follow. However, many regulatory and national patient safety entities are working to establish a standardized measurement to enable hospitals to benchmark against similar systems and develop best practices.

For example, the Agency for Healthcare Research and Quality (AHRQ) has made available its Patient Safety Indicators (PSIs), a set of measures that screen for adverse events patients experience as a result of exposure to the healthcare system. These events are considered preventable once certain changes are made at the provider or unit level. Examples of provider-level indicators include but are not limited to accidental puncture or laceration; birth trauma—injury to neonate; complications of anesthesia; and death in low-mortality diagnosis-related groups. Examples of system-level indicators are postoperative wound dehiscence (rupture), select infections due to medical care, and transfusion reaction. These indicators correspond to ICD-10 codes, making them easy for organizations to obtain.

One patient safety indicator becoming prevalent is serious safety events (SSEs). The American Society for Healthcare Risk Management defines SSEs as those events whose measures deviate from generally accepted practice that reach the patient and whose occurrence causes moderate or severe harm or death. Healthcare Performance Improvement (HPI) has developed a serious safety event rate (SSER) metric that is presented as the number of SSEs that occur in a month divided by the number of patient days in that month divided by 10,000. This result can be displayed in graphical terms and monitored over time. HPI works with organizations to establish a baseline SSER and improve patient safety culture through multiple interventions at all levels of the system.

The Joint Commission (2017) now suggests that organizations perform a root cause analysis for any SSE for which the level of harm is severe or results in death. Many organizations now conduct patient safety culture surveys. A number of vendors offer surveys, but the questions posed to staff, physicians, and leadership are similar regardless of the survey company used. The surveys tend to be clinically focused and represent the perceptions of these groups. An important point to remember is that these surveys share a snapshot in time. Any recent events can affect the perceptions of the staff taking the survey. If an SSE occurred in the recent past or a certain response was made by leaders to a number of recent safety issues and events, that influence will be reflected in the results. These surveys need to be recognized as one data point of many in safety culture measurement. A second perception score can be obtained by administering the Safety Organizing Scale (Vogus and Sutcliffe 2007). This instrument may be more helpful as an ongoing data source, as it contains just nine questions. However, the limitation is that it has only been tested on nursing units.

Another potential metric is overall harm. The idea of an overall harm score has been examined by a number of institutions. This type of measure generally takes into account the total number of incidents of preventable harm in an organization. One instrument that measures harm is the Preventable Harm Score at Nationwide

Children's Hospital (Brilli et al. 2013). It includes not only the number of SSEs but also the number of hospital-acquired infections, adverse drug events, non–intensive care unit cardiac arrests, significant surgical complications, significant falls, and other preventable harm (see exhibit 7.1). Some organizations have taken this metric a step further by including employee safety outcomes.

To improve any of these measures, a baseline of each needs to be established. One measure that has been identified for baseline comparisons is incident and event reporting. As an organization works to improve transparency, it should see a continual increase in incident reporting. Reporting this metric at the unit or department level is especially helpful to improving patient safety, as doing so is meaningful for the staff who work in that area. Organizations can expect to see a continual increase in event reporting during the first year, and while the increased reporting may seem to represent increased harm, it is a reflection of the security individuals feel in the attention being paid to their reports. See chapter 6 for specific interventions to improve transparency.

AHRQ (2012) has established steps organizations can take to improve on the defined PSIs:

- Review and synthesize the evidence base and best practices from scientific literature.
- Work with the multiple disciplines and departments involved in the care of surgical patients to redesign care on the basis of best practices, with an emphasis on coordination and collaboration.
- Evaluate information technology solutions.
- Implement performance measurements for improvement and accountability.

These interventions have elements of process improvement and quality improvement methodologies (Bickel et al. 2015). Healthcare boards and executive leaders need to provide teams with adequate expertise and funding to perform this type of improvement work.

Exhibit 7.1: Patient Safety Dashboard—Preventable Harm Index—for Hospital

Preventable Harm Events	Color Coding Target Key			Year-to-Date (YTD) Events			YTD Cost			YTD Excess Length of Stay (LOS)		
	Green (mid-gray)*	Yellow (light gray)	Red (dark gray)	Current YTD	Projected Annualized Rate	Prior Year	Attributable Cost per Occurrence	YTD Cost	Annualized Cost	Increase in LOS per Occurrence	YTD Extra Days	Annualized Extra Days
Hospital-acquired infections												
Catheter-associated urinary tract infection (CAUTI)				9			$896	$8,064	$16,128			
CAUTI bundle compliance												
Central line-associated bloodstream infection (CLABSI)				14			$45,814	$641,396	$1,282,792	10.4	145.6	291.2
CLABSI with methicillin-resistant *Staphylococcus aureus* (MRSA)							$58,614			15.7		
CLABSI bundle compliance												
Ventilator-associated pneumonia (VAP)							$40,144			13.1		
VAP bundle compliance												
Surgical site infection (SSI)				23			$20,785	$290,990	$581,980	11.2	257.6	515.2
SSI with MRSA							$42,300			23.0		
SSI bundle compliance												
Clostridium difficile infections				83			$11,285	$936,655	$1,873,310	3.3	273.9	547.8
TOTAL ESTIMATED COST AND INCREASED LOS									$3,754,210			1354.2

Preventable Harm Events	Color Coding Target Key			Year-to-Date (YTD) Events			YTD Cost			YTD Excess Length of Stay (LOS)		
	Green (mid-gray)*	Yellow (light gray)	Red (dark gray)	Current YTD	Projected Annualized Rate	Prior year	Attributable Cost per Occurrence	YTD Cost	Annualized Cost	Increase in LOS per Occurrence	YTD Extra Days	Annualized Extra Days
Adverse drug events (severity D-I)												
Category D—Error that required monitoring . . . no harm or intervention to prevent harm												
Category E—Error that may have caused temporary harm and required intervention												
Category F—Error that may have caused temporary harm and required hospitalization												
Category G—Error that may have resulted in permanent harm												
Category H—Error that required intervention to save life												
Category I—Error that may have resulted in death												
Non-ICU cardiac arrests												
List nursing units to identify trends												
Significant complications after surgery												
Unplanned return to surgery within 7 days												
Unexpected death following surgery												
Serious falls												
Fall with fracture												
Fall with laceration requiring sutures												
Fall with loss of consciousness requiring CT scan												
Patient safety indicators (PSIs) not included elsewhere (see dashboard for ind. rates)												
PSI 2-27												
PSI 90 subset												
Serious safety events												
Precursor events												
TOTAL PATIENTS WITH PREVENTABLE HARM												
Safety culture survey—annual results												

Source: Information from Brilli et al. (2013).
Note: All measures are reported as number of events. Cost data are from 2012.
*No green results are showin in this exhibit.

More important, they must be educated in patient safety science and ensure that proven leadership methods are implemented. For example, rounding to influence safety by leadership is a tactic that includes discussion of a department's metrics, conversations regarding incident reporting and any barriers to holding them, and requests for staff commitment to safety.

To hardwire a culture of error reporting, leaders must respond consistently to reported concerns and barriers so that staff continue to report issues. An organization-level safety leadership committee can serve as a repository for safety metrics and safety dashboards. Unit-level leadership can support safety outcomes by discussing them at unit huddles and at staff meetings and by developing lessons learned on the basis of their metrics in preventable harm. Safety stories and discussions about improvements and process changes also support improvement in safety culture.

Ronald Heifetz has often been quoted as saying, "Attention is the currency of leadership." Attention to safety metrics, outcomes, and stories at all levels of the organization is imperative to making improvements. Leaders need to commit to the development of a standardized approach to their patient safety metrics and make the measures easily accessible throughout the organization and to the board. Once a baseline is in place, the specific interventions described throughout this book will assist organizations along their journey to high reliability.

CHAPTER 8

Lessons-Learned Programs, Safety Alerts, and Intranet Dissemination

KEY COMPONENTS OF patient safety improvement at the organizational level include taking a systems approach to safety and institutionalizing a culture of safety. Learning organizations commit to leadership behavior that supports learning and have processes in place to facilitate learning and encourage engagement among employees.

HROs are learning organizations. Their safety data are visible, available, and understandable. Resources for making improvements on the basis of these data include unit-level expertise to assist in preventing any recurrence (Hines et al. 2008).

A strong lessons-learned program and related processes are important elements of a learning organization. Initially, organizations typically build new safety leadership structures and functions to improve their patient safety culture. As mentioned earlier in the book, developing a culture of transparency increases reporting of incidents and events. Once reporting increases in a sustained manner, however, organizational leaders need to be ready to respond.

Some incidents are simple to address with easy fixes. For example, moving equipment closer to the bedside saves work steps, supports staff, and decreases the chance of a work-around being devised. Many, however, are highly complex and require cause analysis and action planning to assist in prevention of recurrence.

Such complicated incidents are likely to occur in many departments across an organization, so the spreading, or dissemination, of information across an organization is necessary. That dissemination requires the development of a standardized approach. Sharing safety stories and examples of incidents has been identified as one way to spread learnings from unit to unit. It helps create risk awareness in terms of system weaknesses and other risk factors. Similarly, sharing good-catch or near-miss events supports the use of safety behaviors and processes. Patients sharing their stories in person or by videotape can be incredibly powerful. The daily safety huddle or safety check-in is another way to spread learnings throughout the organization. Chapter 15 provides more information on the daily safety check-in process.

Another way organizations can spread information is on their internal website or intranet. Safety metrics, safety stories, lessons learned, and executive blog posts on safety and the current status of safety in the organization are elements of a robust and transparent safety culture.

Disseminating lessons learned among physicians may be more difficult than sharing lessons among units. An important starting point is to ensure that supportive executive leadership is in place, including the chief medical officer or vice president of the medical staff. Physicians should be involved in all levels of implementing changes for improvement to safety culture. Some organizations implement a physician safety leadership team or place physician safety under the purview of a current improvement oversight team or committee. The buy-in demonstrated by these clinicians can then be leveraged to design lessons learned among the physician population. Leaders are cautioned to be mindful of the different physician specialties and structures. Working within current communication processes can assist with successful sharing of information.

Finally, a particular challenge is spreading lessons learned across a hospital system. To do so successfully, first, develop a process by which data can be shared across the entity hospitals and sites. Second, develop formal structures and communication points to support the spread of information and improvement efforts. Third, offer multiple opportunities for peers to interact in formal and informal settings to promote widespread improvement.

At those times that an organization needs to address a safety-critical issue—be it with a process, equipment, or a current-state issue such as a medication used in many different departments—the hospital or health system can develop a stop-the-line approach whereby an issue is identified and staff are empowered to halt the process if the patient is at risk. Then an identified safety specialist ensures that a safety alert about the process is disseminated throughout the organization. Identifying an owner of this dissemination process is essential, as is implementing a standard approach to designating which alerts are shared. Some organizations use the situation–background–assessment–recommendation approach, commonly known as SBAR, to develop the alerts in a prompt, succinct, and standard manner. This communication model has gained popularity in healthcare settings. By not overcommunicating the safety information or making it too complex, the stop-the-line process and related communications are easily recognized and absorbed by staff, physicians, and leaders. SBAR is described in detail in chapter 27.

Events that occur in one hospital can easily occur in another hospital anywhere in the United States. In recognition of this fact, several organizations and agencies, such as the American Hospital Association and state-level hospital associations, have worked to design state, regional, and national communication processes that allow safety-critical information to be spread rapidly across all affected organizations using e-mail alerts and centralized websites. In addition, PSOs allow healthcare organizations to share patient safety data, safety alerts, and improvements. These are generally one-page alerts generated by a healthcare entity that has experienced an error. They include the operational areas affected to help target dissemination at the receiving hospitals (Whitmore 2009). Many states now have PSOs associated with their state healthcare association, which provide alerts to participating healthcare systems.

The Joint Commission's chapter governing patient systems produces sentinel event alerts. It states, "the ultimate purpose of The Joint Commission's accreditation process is to enhance quality of care and patient safety." The Joint Commission reviews the sentinel and serious events reported through its database and generates high-level alerts to its participating hospitals, similar to the safety-critical alerts discussed earlier. The sentinel event alerts are thus another way for organizations to recognize where they may have latent system weaknesses before an event occurs. Organizations can also review sentinel event data, root causes, and event types on The Joint Commission website (www.jointcommission.org).

The Emergency Care Research Institute, a nonprofit organization, is dedicated to bringing the discipline of applied scientific research to discover which medical procedures, devices, drugs, and processes are best for application in healthcare. This organization also provides safety alerts.

Finally, the Food and Drug Administration is a central reporting warehouse for medical device failure and medication and nutrition concerns. It disseminates issues and concerns to all hospitals as it deems necessary.

In reviewing elements of HROs, healthcare providers must come to the conclusion that developing the same level of transparency as HROs and becoming a learning organization are top priorities for viability and success in the future.

Building a strong lessons-learned program has been difficult for many organizations but is an important step to becoming highly reliable. Commitment to building both structures and standardized functions for success must be exhibited by the executive leadership of the organization. Building partnerships through state and national PSOs while participating with regulatory organizations can be a first step.

PART III

POSITIONS AND NEW ROLES

CHAPTER 9

New Safety Roles: From the Board to the Front Line

EVERY LEVEL OF a high-reliability organization needs to be aligned with safety as a core value. This broadened agenda requires roles to change and new practices to be adopted. From the board of trustees to frontline staff, the new tactics need to be understood and implemented if outcomes in patient and employee safety are to improve.

To engage all levels of the organization, first, leaders must identify the safety issues that the organization is experiencing. Patient safety stories can bring to staff, management, and board members a realization of the acuteness of an issue. Another tactic for engagement is to provide the organization's patient safety data in a way that is meaningful and relatable to each audience. A third tool, particularly effective for all levels of leadership, is the implementation of just-culture processes. (See chapter 31 for details on building a just culture and the use of just culture algorithms to support high reliability.)

BOARDS AND EXECUTIVE LEADERSHIP

Hospital boards expect their organizations to provide safe, high-quality, compassionate care. With increasingly transparent patient outcomes and with payers reimbursing for performance rather than volume, boards and executive leadership must develop high-reliability methods. Quality improvement and reliability experts recommend that boards put patient safety and harm reduction at the heart of their strategic plans. Furthermore, they suggest carrying out that vision by (1) motivating their management team and clinical staff financially to achieve quality improvement and (2) devoting the resources needed to achieve that vision (Botwinick, Bisognano, and Haraden 2006). The process begins with the board having a comprehensive understanding of patient safety and the resources required to effect change in outcomes.

While improving patient safety is a moral imperative, it also affects an organization's bottom line. Safety events can increase a patient's stay, result in a poor patient experience, and lead to expenditures related to litigation. In addition, occurrences of sentinel events can have secondary costs in the form of employee turnover.

Similar to patient safety, ensuring the safety of employees has a moral as well as financial component. The cost to the organization of lapses in employee safety can manifest in lost productivity, increased turnover, and lack of staff engagement. To keep the board informed and accountable, the organization's leadership needs to provide it with safety-related metrics accompanied by patient and employee safety stories.

Rounding

Whether conducting rounds for safety, rounding to influence, Patient Safety Leadership WalkRounds (IHI and Frankel 2017), or another rounding method, the regular, intentional practice of visiting patient care areas is an approach that both board members and executive leaders can take to support patient and employee safety. Rounding sessions are informal gatherings during which board members and executive leaders go to the units or departments and discuss specific concerns about patient safety with staff and physicians. Initially, staff may feel intimidated; however, that feeling decreases over time as the rounding continues and unit-level issues are addressed. Rounding enables the board members and executive leaders to telegraph the organization's values, mission, and strategies for improving patient outcomes in safety and to demonstrate a caring attitude toward staff. It is also a way to support a flattening of the hierarchy in an organization.

Directors and managers can benefit from rounding in their areas for safety on a regular basis as well. Rounding represents an opportunity for leaders to encourage reporting of incidents and events. Furthermore, this exercise in leadership drives accountability to develop and implement cause analysis programs (discussed in the next section) because the board and senior leadership participate in the analysis process and communicate to staff any improvements to be put in place. In turn, directors and managers can communicate information to the board during rounds, including system-level work to improve outcomes, lessons learned from unit or departmental safety events and incidents, current trends in unit or departmental incidents, and activities to reinforce safety tools and behaviors.

Rounding also demonstrates the importance of support for ongoing education in safety and high-reliability methods to the organization. Here again, relating safety stories is a compelling tactic, as using a unit's own safety stories and safety data to highlight issues engages staff and enables them to understand the value of the tools and education.

Implementing Cause Analysis

Executive leadership can also fulfill the vision of improving safety outcomes by sponsoring cause analysis improvements. Chapter 13 discusses the development and implementation of cause analysis programs. In terms of the role of the executive discussed here, it is to be a highly engaged sponsor in these processes. He or she is charged with ensuring that the care teams are able to make improvements in a timely fashion and that these improvements are sustainable. By its nature, the complexity of healthcare means that the actions to improve system processes also must be complex. Executive leadership is imperative to correcting systemic concerns.

As a valuable by-product of championing cause analysis, executives' engagement and support validate the notion of the organization as a system of continual learning and improvement.

Educating Staff with Safety Data

As mentioned, providing patient safety data to the unit in a relatable manner engages staff. Sharing these data during unit-level huddles or by posting them on briefing boards is one way to provide data and feedback. Disseminating lessons learned, conducting safety data staff meetings, and publishing staff newsletters containing safety data and stories also support this education effort. Resourcing and staffing unit-level safety experts or safety mentors for peer-to-peer support and education is a helpful approach as well. (See chapter 9 for details on developing and implementing programs that encourage staff-level support.)

CLINICAL AND FRONTLINE STAFF

Physicians and staff can also be leaders in safety. A key factor in their development as safety leaders is making sure they are knowledgeable about both the patient safety stories related to events that occur in their area and the safety metrics for their units. Having this information enables them to provide peer support during and after safety incidents and while implementing safety improvements.

Another crucial component of promoting staff and physician safety leadership is an emphasis on staff's use of safety tools and behaviors and on their accountability for the work involved in improving safety. Some organizations highlight the need to adopt safety tools and behaviors by offering financial incentives to staff and physicians through annual reviews, contracting, and bonus programs. Finally, engaging physicians and staff in the development of patient safety improvements, cause analysis teams, and feedback mechanisms can support improvements in outcomes.

Without a commitment to patient and employee safety from all levels of an organization's leadership, outcomes will remain stagnant. Developing and widely sharing an overarching theme of high reliability for patient safety, employee safety, quality, and patient experience enable leadership to transform the organization. A strategic plan that includes the specific tactics discussed throughout this book provides a road map for leadership to high reliability. Furthermore, embracing a culture of safety and accountability, along with continuous learning and attention to the work, can frame the opportunity to improve.

CHAPTER 10

Unit-Based Safety Experts

BUILDING A CULTURE of safety is imperative on the road to becoming a high-reliability organization. A culture encapsulates the prevalent beliefs of a particular society, group, place, or time. It can also be defined as a way of thinking, behaving, or working that pervades a place or an organization. Both definitions include the notion of society or group and of thinking or behaving.

Humans are influenced by those around them. To build a safe culture for our patients and ourselves, peer attention and interaction can support positive change in outcomes.

In high-reliability organizations, the placement of unit-based safety experts (UBSE) is seen as a primary way to achieve a safety culture. Also known as safety mentors, safety coaches, and safety observers, such positions—and leadership's support of them—demonstrate to staff and physicians the importance of safety to the organization. Anyone at any level of the organization can serve as a UBSE, as these are not positions that are necessarily chosen by leadership but rather are filled by individuals who have a keen interest in and passion for the work. Typically, UBSEs spend five to ten hours per month performing peer safety activities, and their salaries are generally absorbed in the unit's budget.

Physicians can also become UBSEs. They may either participate on the staff UBSE committee or have a separate committee structure. Physician UBSEs are educated and trained in the peer safety expert efforts similar to staff UBSEs, with adaptations for working in the physician community.

Allowing UBSEs, particularly physician UBSEs, dedicated and protected time to perform safety work is important to the program's success. Developing the physician's competency in the work can be rewarding to them in a number of ways. (Chapter 15 discusses developing physicians in improvement and safety work in more depth.)

BENEFITS OF UNIT-BASED SAFETY EXPERTS

Safety behaviors, tools, and tactics are often difficult for individuals to build as habits. UBSEs can be instrumental in helping to reinforce the behaviors and to make the tools and tactics relevant to staff's daily work. Each unit or department has its own cultural norms, and UBSEs contextualize the strategies in a way that resonates with those norms. Some organizations highlight a behavior, tool, or tactic each month and tap UBSEs to design information and education for their unit. Then they observe their peers during the month for the designated strategy and provide feedback. Senior leaders can benefit from these observations by reviewing the data collected in documenting the observations as an organizational snapshot.

At first, staff or physicians may feel uneasy providing feedback to their peers. The introduction of scripting early in their development of safety expert work can be helpful for overcoming this issue. Other approaches to increasing their comfort level include discussing tips and tricks at committee meetings, emphasizing the identification of systemic barriers, and coaching the UBSEs to recognize opportunities to offer positive feedback for using the behaviors, tools, and tactics.

A leading cause of patient safety events is the presence of poorly designed teams that are unable to communicate. To begin addressing this issue on a care unit, the organization's patient safety program leader might convene the UBSEs and provide formal education on the functioning of teams and expert-level teamwork. Together, they might then establish parameters for the observation portion of the peer safety expert work to be performed. These observations could include cultural elements, such as pleasantness, respectfulness, and engagement; structural elements, such as briefing, debriefing, closed-loop communication, repeat-backs, and clarifying questions; and an assessment of the current state of operations and other factors: patient volume and acuity, staffing levels, staffing expertise, and so on. Likert-type scales can be used for collecting and correlating data, and subjective data may be added to the observation data using the teamwork questions from the safety culture surveys available from Press Gainey or the Agency for Healthcare Research and Quality or from application of the Safety Organizing Scale.

The observations are intended to determine the degree to which the peers are performing the safety behaviors. If they are not performing them, or are performing them incorrectly, the UBSE and unit leader might develop examples of how and when to use the behaviors. They also might provide examples of errors that have occurred on their units when the safety behaviors are not adopted.

ESTABLISHING A SAFETY EXPERT PROGRAM

The first step in developing a UBSE program is to create a position description. It defines the role and functions for supporting the patient safety culture change through observation and feedback of patient safety habits and processes. Responsibilities and the reporting structure are delineated in the position description, whereby the UBSE is assigned to assist in communicating safety issues, lessons learned from events, and how safety tools and tactics address these issues, and reports to both the unit leadership and safety leadership structure. (Chapter 12 discusses the roles of the safety director and managers.)

Once a position description is defined, the positions are filled for each unit. The UBSEs then are formed in a committee structure for training and education. Education can include discussions of the position description and expectations, safety stories from the organization, the elements of high reliability, current safety efforts, information on how to be an expert observer, discussions about positive feedback, and continuous learning and loop closure for resolving issues. It should also include ample time for questions and feedback. During the education of the UBSE committee, the organization can learn from the UBSEs about current safety trends and concerns.

Beyond the initial training phase, ongoing monthly committee meetings are held by the patient safety program leader, which help keep the UBSEs on track toward fulfilling their roles as defined in the position description. Agenda items for these meetings may include recognition for the work being performed by UBSEs, current organizational trends in safety emerging from the literature or benchmark organizations, guidance regarding areas on which to concentrate their energies for the next month, professional development for the UBSEs, and discussion and feedback on specific activities taking place across the units or departments.

One topic of particular interest for enhancing the contributions of both staff and physician UBSEs is human factors in healthcare. Human factors at play in care delivery are workload; physical ergonomics; cognitive ergonomics, such as time pressures and decision-making processes; and macro-ergonomics, such as teamwork and design efforts (e.g., forcing functions that do not allow errors to occur). The study of human factors provides useful insight for UBSEs as they return to their areas with a mind-set of high reliability. (Chapter 19 provides more detail on mistake proofing and human factors engineering.)

UBSEs are not widely used or highly integrated in patient safety culture improvement efforts, but they can be effective. Peer coaching and checking in a structured program offer high energy and support for change over time. As a program is developed, executive leaders can support it by freeing up the resources needed for safety experts and the UBSE program to flourish.

CHAPTER 11

Getting Physicians on Board: Six Steps to Physician Engagement[1]

SOME OF THE most successful quality leaders are those who have mastered physician engagement. But working with physicians in a positive and collaborative manner eludes many healthcare executives and physician leaders.

Physicians influence 85 percent of patient outcomes based on the decisions they make and the orders they write. Thus, physician engagement is critical to one's success as a safety leader. The ability to partner with these colleagues in a collaborative, collegial, respectful, and honest way is the difference between a great safety program and a mediocre one.

PHYSICIAN CULTURE

The road to physician engagement starts with learning about physician culture—their norms, their values, and the issues and goals important to physicians as a group.

In fact, the ability to engage with any group requires insight into its culture. Knowledge of a group's ideas, customs, and behavioral norms provides the foundation for an engagement plan.

Exhibit 11.1 lists 16 characteristics of physician culture. This list bears study, as integrating even a handful of the traits into one's daily work can lead to improved relationships with physicians and an enhanced ability to engage them in any number of endeavors. In this chapter, we consider six of the most useful for authentic physician engagement.

Exhibit 11.1: Characteristics and Beliefs of Physicians Working in a Physician Culture

1. The welfare of the patient is the number one concern.
2. The quality of care provided is paramount.
3. Physicians are captain of the ship.
4. They function independently and autonomously.
5. Teamwork is fine, but they are in charge.
6. Their way is the only way because they learned from a master.
7. They are the problem solvers.
8. They must compete with each other.
9. They love involvement and expect to be involved.
10. They do not tolerate being embarrassed.
11. They are taught to be aggressive.
12. They are allowed to indulge their strong egos.
13. They enjoy engaging in lively debates.
14. Their approach to practicing medicine is data driven and evidence based.
15. They want a functional, efficient workshop for their work environment.
16. Healthcare is a caste system—if you're not in "the club."

Source: Adapted from Byrnes (2015a).

PATIENT WELFARE IS TOP OF MIND

Quality and safety are primary concerns of virtually all physicians. They are taught that their job is to ensure that high-quality and safe care is delivered to every patient, every day. Thus, asking physicians to help with quality and safety projects is a clear path to engaging them.

Try this approach: "Hi, Dr. Jones. I need to ask for your help to improve care for our surgical patients. Your expertise is critical in getting this done right. Will you help me?" These three straightforward sentences leverage characteristics 2, 7, and 9, as well as the top trait, in exhibit 11.1. This approach can be used to bring together competing groups of physicians, competing health plan medical directors, even competing hospitals—including their CEOs—to work on quality and safety because the quality/safety discussion is neutral territory and a common interest in the physician culture and thus an easy topic to rally around.

PHYSICIANS ARE PROBLEM SOLVERS

Physicians solve patients' problems and deliver treatments or cures. It is an admirable trait, and one that can be leveraged in improvement work. Pose this query to any physician leader: "Dr. Jones, I have a problem and need your help. Can you help me fix (state your problem)?" Frequently, the response will be, "Sure, tell me more."

For every quality improvement project and every patient safety initiative, leaders and staff are solving problems. Sometimes it requires streamlining a process, standardizing order sets, or hardwiring evidence-based medicine into the culture. Whatever the project, this is one of the physician characteristics to tap for fostering engagement.

PHYSICIANS ARE COMPETITIVE

If any silver bullets exist in achieving physician engagement, competitiveness is one of them. It remains an undeniable trait among physicians and is often used to gain otherwise unachievable improvements in error rates and patient outcomes.

Physicians were selected by medical school admission committees in part for their competitiveness. To complete medical school, they must have been vigorous competitors, and they had to have been even better competitors to make it through residency. This competitive nature can explain much of the behavior they exhibit, and a leader's ability to tap into it can lead to meaningful and productive collaboration.

The trait of competitiveness comes into play particularly when data are involved—and even more so if the data concern a physician's personal performance. Often, all that is needed to nudge a physician to improvement is to distribute physician-level performance metrics to a group of doctors and stand back. The public accessibility of the data to peers reliably triggers a competitive urge to improve and best their colleagues' performance—typically within one measurement cycle.

One key to leveraging this attribute on a regular basis is to do so in the spirit of friendly competition. The physicians may be competing against each other, but they are also helping and collaborating with each other to improve care.

Data may also be used to underpin friendly competition among separate groups, such as physicians, nurses, pharmacists, CEOs, and hospital boards. Consider this physician attribute when designing a quality or safety initiative and, if it makes sense, work it into the design framework by presenting data that compare everyone to each other or to a common goal.

PHYSICIANS LOVE INVOLVEMENT

Physicians want to be involved in decisions that affect them, their patients, their hospitals, or their medical group. That desire includes being part of quality improvement teams.

Say you are working to improve outcomes and error rates in total joint replacement. You and your administrator colleagues assume the physicians are too busy to be involved at the beginning of the project, so your team sets out to redesign some care pathways without their input.

This is one of the most common mistakes made in quality and safety programs. Yes, physicians are busy, but they make time for any endeavor they feel is important, particularly those that affect their patients or their practice. Not only do they resent having things "done to them," but they also tend to genuinely enjoy being involved in decision making.

If physicians are unavailable to participate, they place their trust in a well-respected peer to represent their interests and viewpoints. Always invite them to participate. They will make excellent contributions to your effort.

PHYSICIANS DO NOT TOLERATE EMBARRASSMENT

No one likes to be embarrassed, including physicians. During meetings or conversations that involve physician profiles, be particularly conscious about how the data are presented and any comments about them are stated. One helpful tactic is to rehearse what you plan to say. Avoid embarrassing a physician—especially in public, but also in private—because recovery of the damaged relationship may take months or years, seriously derailing engagement efforts.

PHYSICIANS ARE DATA DRIVEN

Physicians are educated as scientists. They are trained in the scientific method, and they are data driven. This trait helps explain why providing feedback to physicians on their performance is so successful in moving them toward improvement of outcomes, complication rates, readmission rates, mortality rates, or error rates.

As stated at the outset of this chapter, having an in-depth understanding of physician culture is beyond important to hospital–physician relations—it is the key to physician engagement in safety and quality efforts.

NOTE

1. Portions of this chapter have been adapted from Byrnes (2015c).

CHAPTER 12

The Safety Specialist and Other Key Staff[1]

QUALITY DEPARTMENTS ARE frequently understaffed and under-resourced. The absence of a robust quality program results in poor safety and satisfaction outcomes as well as unacceptable levels of quality. High-performing organizations have a quality-driven structure in place that has a comprehensive improvement model at its core (exhibit 12.1). In this chapter, we detail the role and function of the safety specialist position and explore the building of a safety department as a whole.

SAFETY SPECIALIST TRAITS

A well-organized hospital quality department includes staff with several distinct skill sets. Generally, these highly experienced professionals learn the science of quality and safety when they come into the position. Hiring staff with nontraditional backgrounds—that is, individuals with nonclinical backgrounds—can enhance their roles. While specific roles and responsibilities apply to the safety specialist position, all members of the quality department should be educated in safety culture and reliability science so that reliability is integrated into all improvement processes. A typical recommendation for staffing ratios is one safety specialist for every 100 beds.

Exhibit 12.1: Quality Department Organizational Chart

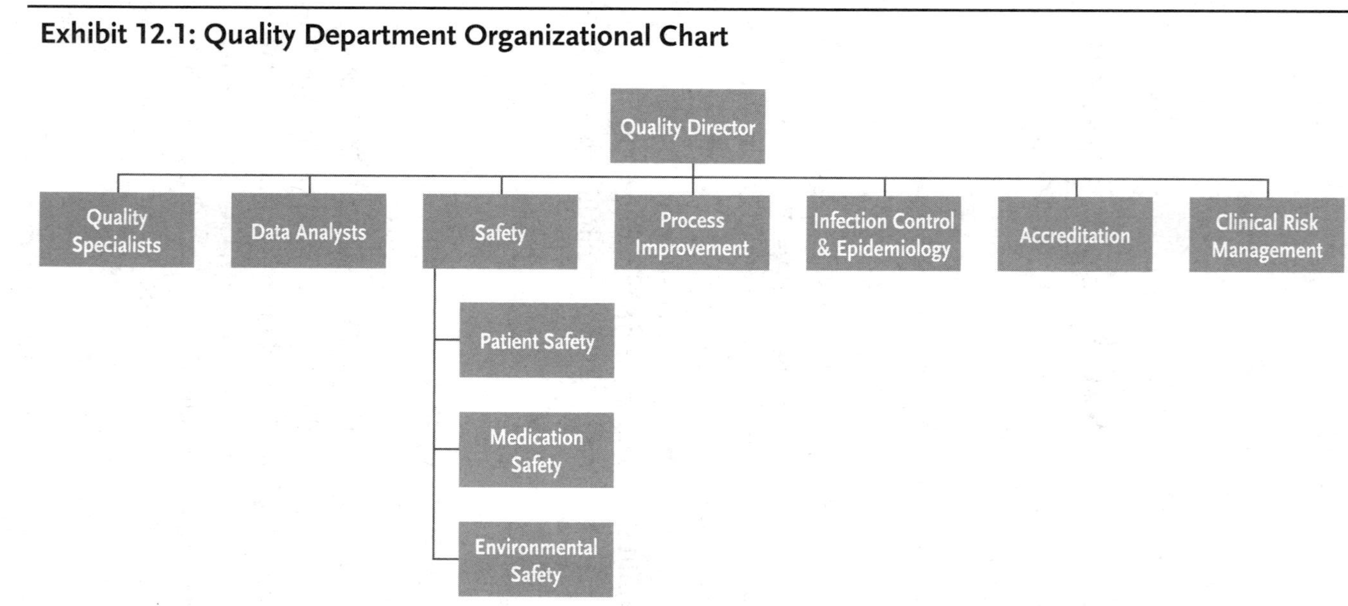

Source: Reprinted with permission from Byrnes (2015c, 133).

The safety specialist role is new to healthcare. Traditionally, ensuring safety in healthcare has been the purview of the environmental safety department, which is regulated by state health departments and accrediting bodies such as The Joint Commission. Now, however, the importance of the safety specialist position to organizations is evidenced by its influence on improving outcomes over time rather than addressing safety events individually as they occur.

Safety culture improvement takes place when the correct structures and tactics are implemented as described throughout this book. As important is the individual who is charged with implementing them. The safety specialist should be highly credible and visible, and one of the organization's best-performing and brightest professionals—an employee whom other departments wish they had on staff. Other key traits possessed by the ideal safety specialist are as follows:

- Optimistic
- Equipped to face any challenge or difficult situation
- Willing to discuss topics or issues that are unpopular
- Adept at educating staff about safety in terms of managing the chain of command—and willing to do so as well
- Self-possessed and driven by passion for the work
- Connected to the deeper purpose of keeping patients safe from harm
- Competitive, often aiming for the organization's care to be the very best in the nation
- Lifelong learner who keeps track of trends that prove to enhance safety, quality, and satisfaction outcomes

Employee Safety Specialist Role

Employee safety is discussed in detail in chapter 5. Staffing for the employee safety specialist role should essentially mirror the patient safety specialist role described earlier. Traditionally, staff in this position worked in the organization's employee health department. Now, however, organizations are applying the science of safety to issues of employee safety and are integrating the role into the quality department's safety division.

In small organizations, the safety specialist may oversee both patient and employee safety. By practicing comprehensive safety science standards, this approach allows such organizations to apply the same tactics to prevent errors and harm in team members.

OTHER KEY SAFETY STAFF

Infection Preventionist

Infection prevention is a section of the quality department that works hand in hand with the safety specialists. Infection preventionists are physicians, nurses, and epidemiologists trained in the prevention, detection, and control of infections. They are vital to the work of preventing hospital-acquired conditions such as central line infections and ventilator-associated pneumonia.

In addition, infection preventionists apply high-reliability principles to train peer safety experts, such as UBSEs, in tactics such as peer checking (e.g., speaking up when another team member misses an opportunity to wash his or her hands) to improve the infection outcomes for the organization. Infection prevention professionals should also be highly trained in cause analysis principles to be able to identify the root causes of upward trends in infection rates. (Cause analysis is discussed in depth in chapter 13.)

Medication Safety Officer

A major cause of injury to patients is medication error. To help reduce the incidence of medication errors, many organizations now have a medication safety officer, typically a staff pharmacist trained in safety science. The individual in this role conducts reviews and monitors trends of medication errors in the organization; studies the human factors surrounding technology, such as electronic health records and smart IV pumps; and reviews all medication processes, policies, procedures, and guidelines. The medication safety officer works closely with a variety of departments to address concerns related to administering high-risk, low-volume medications. He or she is also knowledgeable about recommendations for medication administration from agencies such as the Institute for Safe Medication Practices, the US Food and Drug Administration, and The Joint Commission.

SAFETY SPECIALIST ROLES AND OTHER ORGANIZATIONAL AREAS

As with patient and employee safety specialists, the individuals who work in the infection preventionist and medication safety officer roles should be capable of getting along well with others. These types of so-called soft skills allow them to develop effective working relationships with physicians and nursing leaders and manage difficult teams and personalities. They often find themselves facilitating discussions that include making major process changes to address gaps in the system of care. They need to serve as objective observers for the organization to suggest adjustments to protocols.

Patient safety specialists, employee safety specialists, medication safety officers, and infection prevention specialists can all benefit from training in clinical quality improvement, project management, team facilitation, and Lean or Six Sigma process improvement methods. Training in root cause, apparent cause, and common cause analysis is also helpful. With this skill set, they are well positioned to work with the organization's project management office or process improvement personnel on safety-specific improvement initiatives.

Organizations that have the capability to make major improvements in error prevention operate safety and quality departments that are closely aligned with the risk management department. All the safety specialist roles discussed in this chapter work closely with risk management professionals, who review incidents and errors as they occur. Healthcare organizations are moving away from traditional reactive risk management toward enterprise risk management. Enterprise risk management is a business discipline that addresses all risks and seeks to manage their impact in a way that supports the strategic achievement of an organization's objectives. Once the risks are identified, risk management professionals can engage their safety and quality colleagues to assist with designing improvement initiatives. With incidents and errors that have already occurred, this same group can perform cause analysis and action planning to prevent recurrence.

Ultimately, the difference between high quality and poor, or even average, quality is the people who do the work. Just as senior leaders aggressively manage the financial performance of their organizations, they must apply that same aggressiveness to manage quality and safety performance. Reimbursement for performance will require organizations to diligently improve their performance. Those organizations in turn will need dedicated staff with contemporary skills that match today's national agenda.

NOTE

1. Portions of this chapter have been adapted from Byrnes (2015c).

PART IV

TOOLS

CHAPTER 13

Root Cause, Apparent Cause, and Common Cause Analysis

ALTHOUGH CAUSE ANALYSIS in healthcare has resulted in inconsistent outcomes, a strong cause analysis program is integral to the success of a high-reliability organization.

The goal of cause analysis is to identify the causes of an incident or event and build in new or improved processes so that the incident or event does not recur, thereby improving patient outcomes.

Healthcare has traditionally applied training and education to fix problems, but those problems are often caused not by a lack of knowledge but rather by an issue with the system or process. This misapplied education is a main reason cause analysis has not consistently supported the correction of healthcare error events. This chapter identifies the qualities of an efficient, effective, and comprehensive cause analysis program for healthcare.

ROOT CAUSE ANALYSIS

Root cause analysis (RCA) is the most frequently discussed cause analysis tool. The Joint Commission (2013) describes RCA as the entire investigative and corrective action process following a sentinel event, and the accrediting body requires that events of moderate temporary harm or above undergo RCA.

Most organizations agree that events of severe, permanent harm or death require an RCA. To support their efforts, the National Patient Safety Foundation (2015) released a white paper titled *RCA²: Improving Root Cause Analyses and Actions to Prevent Harm.* It encourages hospitals to put as much energy into planning prior to an event as they put into the investigation. One tactic is to develop a process for classifying events and then prioritize the events for the appropriate level of analysis.

RCA Investigations

Event investigation is generally led by the risk management department to ensure that steps are taken to protect the organization from a legal standpoint. At the onset of an investigation, the risk manager notifies the team charged with classifying the event, which helps determine the type of event analysis to pursue, if any.

If an RCA is warranted, an executive sponsor is identified to oversee the process. The role of the executive sponsor includes the following responsibilities (NPSF 2015):

- Ensure that the immediate situation is safe (e.g., removing equipment, ensuring that staff or physicians are safe to continue caring for patients, determining whether the event could occur at any moment in any other areas).
- Meet with the RCA team—typically made up of five to six individuals—to discuss and agree on the investigation's scope.
- Establish priorities regarding which elements of the action plan are completed first.
- Allocate resources.
- Remove any barriers to investigations or to planning actions that will prevent the error or incident from recurring.

- Communicate findings and improvements to the rest of the executive team.
- Take accountability for the entire process.

RCA teams may differ from organization to organization. A typical RCA team includes risk management personnel, a safety specialist, unit-level leadership, physician leadership, a unit-based subject matter expert, and a quality or performance improvement specialist.

Once the investigation is deemed to be complete, the RCA team and executive sponsor meet to determine any gaps in the standards of care or accepted processes. From there, an action plan is developed for effecting changes to avoid recurrence.

As with any change in processes, policies, or procedures, the effectiveness of a safety-related change needs to be audited and adjusted, in much the same way as the Plan, Do, Study, Act (PDSA) cycle is applied to process improvement initiatives. The resulting action plan should be reviewed at regular intervals, such as every 30 days, by the executive sponsor. The executive sponsor uses these reviews to become aware of any barriers to implementing the change.

The executive sponsor, in conjunction with unit and physician leadership, must take accountability for the successful implementation of safety-related changes, rather than risk management personnel or safety or quality specialists. The roles of the risk management, safety, and quality areas are to support and facilitate the process as a whole, not be responsible for the outcomes.

RCAs usually take 35 to 40 hours to complete. An example of an RCA process is shown in exhibit 13.1.

Barriers to Effective Root Cause Analysis

Incomplete investigations are often the most significant deterrent to an effective RCA. To avoid this issue, the team charged with

Exhibit 13.1: Sample RCA Process

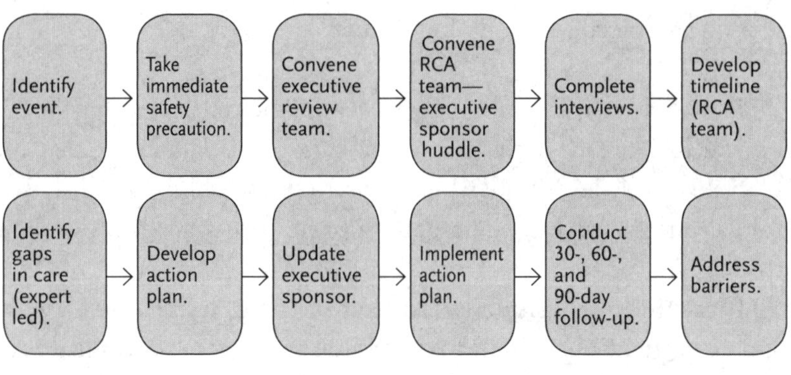

conducting RCAs should develop a consistent investigative approach. Employing a process improvement technique called the 5 whys is one way to ensure that the RCA team takes the investigation through to its end. Developed by Sakichi Toyoda, founder of the Toyota Motor Company, the 5 whys is an interrogative strategy used to explore the cause-and-effect relationships underlying a particular problem. The primary goal of the technique is to determine the root cause of a defect or problem by repeating the question *Why?* where each question's answer forms the basis of the next question. The *5* in the name derives from an empirical observation of the number of iterations typically required to resolve problems.

This technique can be helpful in performing the investigative portion of the RCA, as often healthcare personnel jump right into an action plan without understanding the problem. Using 5 whys when investigating any event provides the information needed to determine the cause or causes accurately.

APPARENT CAUSE ANALYSIS

Apparent cause analysis (ACA) is relatively new to healthcare. An ACA is a limited investigation of an event that is often performed in lieu of an RCA for less significant events. ACAs are expected to identify corrective actions and collect information necessary to support future common cause analysis (CCA) (discussed in the next section). As with an RCA, an ACA helps address any immediate safety issues at the time of the event. ACAs do not generally have an executive sponsor but are owned at the unit leadership level. In addition, instead of a five- to six-person team, ACAs are conducted by one or two people. The goal is to learn who did what and why. Best practice for ACAs is to have unit-level teams lead the analysis with support from the risk management team and the safety specialist, who is ultimately responsible for ACA outcomes. Finally, ACAs should take two to four hours to perform, as opposed to the approximately 35 to 40 hours spent conducting an RCA.

The ACA process is similar to RCA in that the team investigates the issue, determines the gaps, and develops an action plan to address those gaps. Unit-level leaders sponsor and support the changes, and they audit the outcomes to ensure that the changes in fact improve the safety issue and are sustained.

COMMON CAUSE ANALYSIS

CCA is performed to determine the common causes of the events across an organization (Clapper and Crea 2010). An important notion for understanding the difference between RCA and CCA is to think of CCA in terms of causes and not outcomes.

Organizations view repeat events as cause analysis failures. The reality is that an organization can experience, for example, two cases of retained sponges from two completely different causes. Another scenario is to experience one case of a retained sponge and another case of delayed medication administration where the causes are the same. Such examples demonstrate the value of the 5 whys technique in CCA investigations.

Furthermore, the gaps in care identified by RCAs and ACAs are coded or trended, facilitating the identification of common causes among the events by the safety specialist. Coding can be broken down into individual and system errors, then further separated into the types of errors as determined by the investigation.

THE EMERGING PATIENT ROLE IN CAUSE ANALYSIS

Many organizations have begun to integrate the participation of patients and patient families in their cause analysis processes. While an organization must be mindful of legal and psychological issues related to this practice, patients and families have a unique frame of reference and can provide feedback that cannot be obtained through team member interviews or in case review. Some organizations that retain family representatives in paid positions or that seat patient or family advisory councils ask these representatives to participate in cause analysis. Their involvement can help the family recover following an event and assist the organization in rebuilding the community's trust in addition to providing the hospital or health system with valuable input.

Cause analysis has become a necessary tool for building high reliability. An organized and standardized approach is essential to efficient and effective cause analysis, and executives can assist the entire process by making it transparent and promoting it as an organizational priority. One positive by-product of internal cause analysis training is the spreading of the expertise across the organization.

CHAPTER 14

Error Prevention Behaviors: Making It Stick

Craig Clapper, chief knowledge officer at Healthcare Performance Improvement, has stated that building an environment toward high reliability requires more tools and fewer rules. These tools include a set of error prevention behaviors used 100 percent of the time by 100 percent of the staff and physicians. These are relatively simple behaviors or tactics, but while educating everyone about them may not be difficult, adopting and maintaining them at the 100 percent level can be.

Error prevention behaviors are designed to address the way the mind works. Human error is the inadvertent failure to do other than what should have been done. Error prevention behaviors are intended to overcome the mind-set or inclinations that lead to a slip, lapse, or mistake. Error prevention behaviors and their related tools and functions are discussed throughout the book; this chapter focuses on how to implement and sustain them.

INTRODUCING ERROR PREVENTION BEHAVIORS

Organizations aiming to change their patient safety culture must first make safety an organizational value, in part by placing it as a priority in the strategic plan. In introducing the strategies and tactics outlined in this book, an effective approach is to build the safety culture on patient safety stories of incidents that have occurred in the organization; the same is true for error prevention strategies. Using these stories, patient safety facilitators and educators help staff and physicians understand the "why" underlying the behaviors they are asked to integrate into daily practice.

The first step in introducing error prevention behaviors is consistent education about them provided to all board members, staff, leaders, and physicians. This education is best received when modified for the audience. For example, a presentation of the information to the board is modified to assist its members in understanding why the organization is asking the staff to adopt these behaviors and how implementation of the program affects patient outcomes. Similarly, error prevention strategies presented to clinical areas may vary from those offered to support services departments. However, the content of the education should be consistent; for example, it should be presented with a safety story about an error that occurred in the organization.

Second, the error prevention program leaders provide information about the nationwide concerns, data, and stories related to patient and employee safety. One small but effective tactic in this step is to pause briefly to allow the audience to absorb the information and to gauge attendees' reactions. Often, staff, and even physicians and board members, are unaware of the national scale of the safety problem.

The third step takes place once the organization's board, clinical staff, and support staff have learned and understood the why of error prevention behavior training and implementation. It involves teaching, in an objective way, the actions they can take and strategies they can adopt as individuals to prevent errors. (Chapter 34 describes a sample timeline and plan for providing the types of education discussed here and elsewhere in the book.)

Finally, a best practice for providing education on safety behaviors is to use simulation. This approach is most effective when presented during in-person sessions with trainers, facilitators, and educators who have received extensive safety science education as well as training in the specific content of the session topic.

One way organizations use simulation in training is to present videos demonstrating examples of the behaviors—both the incorrect and correct ways to use them. Following the video presentation, the educators facilitate role-play simulation of the behaviors.

If staff members leave a training session with questions or discomfort about next steps, the conversation must be continued, perhaps by having staff perform the scenario a second time with the aid of cues or feedback. Debriefing with the group following a role-playing simulation on how it felt to take part in the error, what participants noticed as the situation unfolded, and how they might apply the learning in their area also helps solidify the behavior.

Another way simulation can be used to train for error prevention behaviors, for those organizations that have a well-developed simulation or team training program, is to repeat simulations on an ongoing basis. Patient safety specialists and trainers attend these simulations and identify a variety of situations in which the behaviors can be used.

Organizations with robust simulation or training programs can take the education further by adding simulation to the root cause and apparent cause analysis processes. Simulation during cause analysis takes place in the simulation laboratory or as a patient safety event is unfolding. These just-in-time simulations can be valuable in identifying the system weaknesses and addressing them in real (or near-real) time. (Simulation for patient safety is discussed in detail in chapter 17.)

HARDWIRING ERROR PREVENTION

Education and simulation may be seen as the easy part. More difficult is embedding these behaviors as habits and sustaining the change. One way to begin is to highlight one behavior or tool per month for all areas of the organization. Building the habit of exercising several behaviors at once can be overwhelming. Taking one at a time, especially early on in the work, can help all members of the organization hardwire their individual knowledge and use of the behavior.

The monthly highlight can be presented as part of a safety discussion at the beginning of all meetings, daily huddles, staff meetings, or unit-based communications about lessons learned; displayed on performance boards; or distributed via e-mail or the internal website. Encouraging staff to discuss how they used the behavior is an effective way to spread adoption via peer-to-peer communication. Another approach is to hold competitions in the use of the behavior. However an organization promotes error prevention behaviors, ongoing and consistent information regarding the behaviors keeps them at the forefront of thought for all its members (Griffith 2010).

The leaders of an organization must understand and be able to speak to all the error prevention techniques that have been adopted as part of the patient safety culture design. When rounding in any department, organizational leaders can engage the staff in discussions of the safety behavior that is being highlighted that month. Similarly, leaders at the department level can reinforce the hardwiring of error prevention behaviors while conducting daily, weekly, or monthly communications with their staff. When a patient safety event occurs, leaders throughout the organization need to communicate about the behaviors that, had they been exercised correctly, could have prevented the error.

Error prevention behaviors are the foundation for building a safe culture. These behaviors are applied in the care of patients, but they are equally important for keeping employees safe as well. Their integration as daily habits helps ensure a zero-incident environment—a goal to which each hospital and health system should aspire.

CHAPTER 15

Situational Awareness, Shift Planning, Daily Check-ins, and Safety Huddles

As HIGH-RELIABILITY ORGANIZATIONS, healthcare entities need to be sensitive to activities or situations (e.g., high census, low-volume or high-risk procedures, new processes or procedures, staffing problems, equipment or medication shortages) that can lead to an increased chance of error. This attention requires leaders to have situational awareness about frontline issues. Throughout all levels of the organization, executives and managers must have current knowledge and understanding about operational issues, the level of risk a situation or activity poses, and potential trends for future risks and consequences. One widely adopted tactic to support situational awareness among leaders is to conduct an organization-wide standup check-in every 24 hours.

ORGANIZATION-WIDE HUDDLES

This practice originated in the nuclear power industry, where each day begins with a plan-of-the-day meeting of plant leaders. In the healthcare organization, this daily safety huddle or check-in is led by a C-suite executive, with the lead executive rotating periodically.

Each department or service line sends a manager or another representative to attend, and each attendee reports back on any issues that arose in the past 24 hours and any high-risk concerns for the upcoming 24 hours (Stockmeier and Clapper 2011). Examples of such issues include the following:

- Implementation of a new process or procedure
- Installation of a new piece of equipment
- IT downtime or major system upgrade
- A scheduled high-risk, low-volume procedure
- A patient presenting with an unusual condition or illness

In this reporting process, special attention needs to be paid to those issues or incidents that can occur in other areas. High-risk issues that can have a major impact on the organization should be assigned to a designated individual for follow-up, with the expectation that he or she will update the group in the next 24 to 48 hours.

The executive leading the daily safety huddle or check-in is responsible for reviewing any barriers the unit leadership encounters in addressing the cause of the risk or event. Many organizations also use the daily huddle to discuss any census, staffing, and throughput issues. Hot spots for the day, such as staffing issues, patients at risk for deterioration, new or infrequent diagnoses or procedures, new technology, and high census, are discussed, and solutions are driven by consensus to ensure the safest approach is taken.

Generally, one attendee takes notes so that issues can be tracked and trended. These notes are sent to the leaders for their review to confirm the details and reinforce action plans. A telephone conference line may be set up for those who cannot attend, especially in large organizations whose leadership is spread out geographically. While this accommodation facilitates wide participation, in-person attendance is strongly encouraged, as a secondary gain from this style of huddle is that the managers get to see each other face-to-face and take part in impromptu discussions, thereby building strong collegial relationships. Executives and department directors should keep track of attendance and follow up with any managers who fail to attend regularly or to send a designee and address any barriers faced in their ability to participate.

DEPARTMENT-LEVEL HUDDLES

At the department or unit level, shift huddles and shift overviews are held with all caregiving staff to help continually build situational awareness. One tool for conducting these huddles is the daily improvement board, from the Lean performance improvement toolbox. A white board is marked to show columns, or swim lanes (see exhibit 15.1). The first lane shows the unit's current state, including census; number of admissions in the past 24 hours; number of discharges anticipated in the next 24 hours; staffing levels; and high-risk, "watcher" patients. (*Watcher* is a term coined by Cincinnati Children's Hospital for patients who need frequent assessment and intervention due to their symptomology [Brady et al. 2013]).

The second lane conveys information on safety, such as issues or incidents experienced in the past 24 hours that all staff need to be aware of; recognition of staff members for good catches; recent safety data, including safety culture survey results; and follow-up regarding concerns about any risks identified earlier by the staff. The fourth lane focuses on the staff and may include staff satisfaction data, additional recognition for staff, and teamwork information and data. The final lane documents data on the patient experience, including patient and family experience survey findings, improvement work related to the patient experience, a featured patient story, and patient feedback and suggestions.

The third lane on the daily improvement board lists quality or process improvement metrics. These measures can include hospital-acquired condition information, progress to date on current PDSA cycles, information about other process improvement work, highlights from the previous 24-hour rounding, and any findings from recent accreditation or regulatory audits.

Exhibit 15.1: Example of a Huddle or Daily Improvement Board

Current State	Safety	Quality/Process Improvement	Staff	Patients and Families
Census: 25	Incidents/issues	HACs CLABSIs: last date 5/25/17	Staff satisfaction survey results	This week's patient story
Admissions: 4	Safety culture survey	Falls: last date 6/1/17	Recognition	Patient experience data
Discharges: 5	Good catches	Rounding feedback:	Staff suggestions	Patient/family feedback
Watchers: Room 204 Room 210	Incident/issue follow-up:			
	Joint Commission visit starts August 1!			

Note: CLABSI = catheter-associated bloodstream infection; HAC = hospital-acquired condition.

Unit-based shift huddles should last approximately 15 minutes and be facilitated by unit leadership. The unit quality improvement specialist and safety specialists can assist by providing much of the data. New information is briefly reviewed, and staff are encouraged to speak up about any concerns or make suggestions for improvement.

The participative nature of the daily shift overview and accompanying documentation on the white board allow all staff who work on the unit to be aware of safety activities and issues. All disciplines should participate in the huddle to further ensure that each member of the team has a good working knowledge of the risks that are present for the upcoming shift. On units that span a large physical area, these huddles may occur in multiple locations. For example, different surgical services staff may huddle in the preoperative area, surgical suite, and recovery area.

LEADERSHIP ROUNDING

Another way to increase situational awareness is through leadership rounding. Rounding to influence behavior is discussed at length elsewhere in the book as a leadership tactic to support high reliability. While this approach is primarily intended to influence staff and physician practice behaviors, it also informs leaders about the pulse and tone of the units. Executives can learn the overall as well as specific concerns of the staff and physicians and uncover barriers to safe care. When these issues are addressed in a timely fashion, staff recognize that the organization supports the staff and that patient and employee safety really is a core value.

When unit-based leaders, including physicians, round on the units, they can become aware of latent, or hidden, system weaknesses as they are voiced by the staff, physicians, and patients and families. If space on the unit's huddle board is dedicated to documenting issues that arise during rounding, a trip to the huddle board following a rounding session can further raise awareness for executives and unit leadership as these issues are addressed by team members. It also serves as a means to recognize staff in real time for providing feedback.

TRANSPARENCY AND A SUPPORTIVE CULTURE

The report *Shining a Light: Safer Healthcare Through Transparency* (Lucian Leape Institute 2015) indicates that three main cultural elements are key to improving transparency among clinicians, CEOs, other leaders, and staff. The first component is a supportive culture in which caregivers can be transparent with and accountable to each other. The second element is a comprehensive set of multidisciplinary processes and forums for reporting, analyzing, sharing, and using safety data for improvement. The final component is the creation of processes to address noncompliance by building accountability practices. (Building accountability practices is discussed in more detail in chapter 31.)

When these cultural elements are present in an organization, each individual feels responsible, accountable, and safe to provide accurate information on departmental issues (Lucian Leape Institute 2015).

Once executives, leaders, physicians, and staff all accept responsibility for discussing their concerns, areas of risk, errors that have occurred, and patient stories, situational awareness has taken hold at the highest level. Rounding, huddle boards, and organization-wide daily safety huddles and check-ins provide comprehensive support for all members of the organization to practice a culture of safety.

CHAPTER 16

Brief and Debrief Huddles for Surgical Care

If you don't know where you're going, you might end up somewhere else.

—Yogi Berra

Communication breakdown is a common root cause in 50% to 70% of sentinel events.

—The Joint Commission

Communication breakdowns can occur during all phases of surgical care—preoperative, operative, and postoperative—and can result in the death, disability, or prolonged length of stay of the patient undergoing surgery (Greenberg et al. 2007). For example, operating room (OR) personnel have reported that a lack of discussion and systematic planning before skin incision begins is common (Bethune et al. 2011).

Furthermore, a study of communication failures in the OR found that poor communication occurs in approximately 30 percent of team exchanges. And nearly a third of such failures lead to increased cognitive load, interrupted routines, and increased tension among caregivers—all of which jeopardize patient safety (Lingard et al. 2004). In the postoperative period, failure to communicate intraoperative events to the postop care team can result in the inappropriate monitoring of patients following surgery; a lack of vigilance for predictable postoperative complications; and medication errors, such as lapses or delays in antibiotic administration or delays in taking preventive measures for patients at risk for deep-vein blood clots.

THE PRE-PROCEDURAL BRIEFING

The preoperative or pre-procedural briefing is a critical safety tool in highly complex industries. Such briefings or huddles facilitate the sharing of critical information and help create an atmosphere of learning and responsibility (Helmreich et al. 2001). In healthcare, huddles also provide an opportunity for members of the care team to coordinate care and to raise safety concerns. Briefings take place shortly before the start of a procedure or at the beginning of the day when all cases are reviewed together. A sample preoperative briefing guide is shown in exhibit 16.1.

History of Huddles

Huddles originated in American football in 1894 with Paul D. Hubbard, the quarterback at Gallaudet University, a premier college for deaf students (Gannon 1981). References to huddles in the medical literature started to appear in 1993, and by the mid-2000s, huddles were in widespread use in healthcare, particularly in ORs, labor and delivery critical care units, and emergency departments.

Exhibit 16.1: Preoperative Briefing Guide[1]

VETERANS HEALTH ADMINISTRATION

Preoperative Briefing Guide for Use in the Operating Room

✓ Read and Verify Checklist, Local Facilities Decide When Checklist Completed.

- ❑ **Patient Name[1-4]**
- ❑ **Social Security #, Birthdate, or Other VA-Approved Identifier[1]**
- ❑ **Names & Roles of Team Members[2]**
- ❑ **Procedure[1-4]**
- ❑ **Surgical Site[1-4]**
  - ❑ Marked or on Wristband
- ❑ **Laterality/Side[1-4]**
- ❑ **Known Allergy[2]**
  - ❑ No
  - ❑ Yes
- ❑ **Anesthesia[2]**
  - ❑ Difficult Airway, Aspiration Risk?
    - ❑ No
    - ❑ Yes
    - ❑ If Yes, Equipment & Assistance Available
    - ❑ Safety Check Completed
    - ❑ Pulse Oximetry
- ❑ **Instruments & Special Equipment[2-4]**
  - ❑ N/A
  - ❑ Yes
- ❑ **Implant(s)[1-4]**
  - ❑ N/A
  - ❑ Yes
  - ❑ If Yes, Specifics

- ❑ **Pertinent Lab Results**
- ❑ **Risk of >500 ml Blood Loss[2,4]**
  - ❑ No
  - ❑ Yes, and adequate IV access and fluids planned, and blood availability confirmed
  - ❑ If Yes,
    - ❑ Type & Screen

    OR
    - ❑ Type & Cross
- ❑ **Prophylactic Antibiotics Given Within 60 Minutes of Incision[2-4]**
  - ❑ Yes
  - ❑ N/A
- ❑ **DVT Prophylaxis[4]**
  - ❑ Yes
  - ❑ N/A
- ❑ **Anticipated Critical Events[2]**
  - ❑ Surgeon
  - ❑ Anesthesia
  - ❑ Nursing
- ❑ **Postop Disposition & Bed Availability[4]**

STOP

TIME OUT!

- ❑ **Name of patient & SS# or birthdate**
- ❑ **Procedure to be performed**
- ❑ **Position**
- ❑ **Consent form checked (patient, procedure, site/side, reason)**
- ❑ **Check that surgical site marked and visible after draping and/or wristband confirmed**
- ❑ **Implant to be used (if applicable)**
- ❑ **Two members confirm imaging studies available, correct, properly labeled, presented**
  - ❑ **Yes**
  - ❑ **N/A**

This checklist contains the elements of the WHO checklist and also includes a sampling of the majority of elements as suggested by frontline OR teams from the VHA. The WHO Surgical Safety Checklist is available at http://www.safesurg.org/uploads/1/0/9/0/1090835/sssl_checklist_finaljun08.pdf

[1]VHA Policy/Directive, [2]WHO Checklist, [3]Joint Commission, [4]Medical Team Training

Source: Adapted from Jain et al. (2015).

Performing the Briefing

Many institutions use a checklist to support preoperative huddles. The checklists speed up the briefing process and, more important, decrease the risk that care team members will forget important aspects of the procedure to take place. Checklists have also been found to significantly improve communication and recall of critical steps, especially in situations where caregivers are performing an emergency procedure, when gathering for a huddle is not possible, such as a STAT cesarean delivery or trauma surgery (Dadiz et al. 2013).

Typical participants in a preoperative huddle include those involved in the patient's care in the OR or procedural area, such as the following:

- The surgeon(s)
- The anesthesia provider(s)
- The OR nurses
- The scrub technicians
- The recovery room nurse(s)
- The patient

Typical information in the preop huddle for an obstetric case could include the following (surgical huddles would be similar in scope):

- Team introductions and roles
- Confirmation of the patient's identity, signed consent forms, medications, and allergies
- Statement of the surgery or procedure to be performed, and marking of the surgical site
- Review of critical and nonroutine steps of the surgery or procedure

- Confirmation of the availability and readiness of implants or special equipment
- Review of pertinent laboratory values
- Statement regarding anticipated blood loss and confirmation of the availability of blood products
- Review of planned anesthetic use and plan for monitoring airway and other anesthetic concerns
- Review of neonatal concerns
- Confirmation of antibiotic administration and dosing
- Review of deep venous thrombosis (DVT) prophylaxis protocol
- Review of postoperative plans and contingencies
- Mention of any additional concerns

THE POSTPROCEDURAL BRIEFING, OR DEBRIEFING

A debriefing is a review that occurs following an operation or a procedure. The goal is to review both negative and positive events that occurred during the case while it is still fresh in the minds of the team members. Debriefing offers an opportunity to identify and promptly address equipment issues, adjust processes, and coordinate care and plan for the ongoing needs of the patient post-procedure.

The use of debriefings in healthcare began at roughly the same time the World Health Organization (2009) introduced its *Guidelines for Safe Surgery*. The guidelines included tools for preop and postop briefings and the Surgical Safety Checklist.

Performing the Debriefing

The postoperative debriefing takes place in the OR during skin closure or immediately after the end of surgery and includes the same team members as participated in the preoperative huddle. A further advisable practice is to include recovery room personnel, either in person or via phone or intercom, to ensure that good handoffs occur during the transition of the patient from one setting to another.

As with the preoperative huddle, a checklist is a helpful aid and includes items such as the following:

- Summary of the procedure, including totals for volume of blood loss, urine output, intravenous fluids used, blood products used, and medications administered
- Labeling of pathologic specimens with correct patient information
- List of activities that went well
- Description of activities that needed to go better
- Mention of any safety concerns
- List of equipment issues and changes for future cases
- Description of efficiency issues
- Postoperative planning, including special monitoring, equipment, and medications required

BENEFITS OF HUDDLES

The benefits of huddles or briefings have been demonstrated in a wide range of surgical and procedural specialties. For example, several studies have shown that huddles result in improved on-time administration of preoperative antibiotics and DVT prophylaxis. They also reduce the number of unanticipated events and near misses in the OR while preventing equipment issues and improving intraoperative workflow (Einav et al. 2010).

Do huddles delay OR start times? In multiple studies, the answer is shown to be no. In fact, preop huddles improve the rate of on-time starts and even contribute to early starts (Ali et al. 2011).

Furthermore, huddles can improve communication between nursing staff and surgeons, between surgeons and anesthesiologists, between obstetricians and neonatologists, and so on. Improved communication is achieved by providing a framework that circumvents the traditional hierarchy or authority gradient in the OR, and by creating dedicated, protected time to share information and ask questions.

Finally, huddles enhance team members' accountability and empowerment, and they enable staff to speak up in what are traditionally intimidating, high-stress environments. This impact is most pronounced for nurses and team members who occupy a lower status in the OR hierarchy. Not surprisingly, the ability of team members and patients to speak up has been identified by organizations such as the Institute of Medicine as a critical step in avoiding adverse events. The huddle facilitates this process because it provides a place and a time whereby all team members are encouraged to raise issues and concerns without judgment.

Benefits of Debriefings

Likewise, postprocedure debriefings consisting of an exchange of information following an operation have demonstrated numerous benefits. The debriefing structure gives the team an opportunity to review what went well and what could have been improved, including discussion of critical events, errors, or mishaps that occurred during the case. Not surprisingly, recent studies have also shown that a lack of postoperative debriefings increases the risk of complications from procedures (Mazzocco et al. 2009).

Debriefings also allow time for reflection, which is a key component of adult learning, suggesting that implementing a postoperative debriefing is likely to elevate the overall performance and effectiveness of OR staff. Finally, the debriefing affords the opportunity to call out accomplishments and commend team members for a job well done. This activity can have a profound impact on morale while it reinforces a sense of teamwork and improved job satisfaction (Hill et al. 2015).

Exhibit 16.2: Emergency Room Debriefing (DISCERN) Document

DO NOT SCAN OR PUT INTO PATIENT CHART—STAPLE TO CODE SHEET AND TURN INTO MEA'S FOLDER

Texas Children's Hospital—Debriefing in Situ Conversation in Emergency Room Now (DISCERN) Form
This info is privileged and confidential purusant to TX Health & Safety Sections 161.031-033,
TX Occupations Code
Section 160.007 &/or TRCP 192.5

ALL patients need this section completed—NURSE **must decide with the doctor whether a debrief is necessary for** EVERY **resuscitation**		**Fill out this section only if debriefing occurs**	**Fill out this section during the debriefing** (Person writing not the person leading debriefing) (Write on the back of form if there is not enough space)
PLACE PATIENT STICKER HERE 1. Date (MM/DD/YY) 2. Physician Team Leader 3. 1° Nurse filling this out: 4. If team leader & 1° nurse together decide not to do a debriefing, state reasoning: (check one box to the right) (skip #4 if doing debrief) 5. Resuscitation Type (check all that apply) 6. Interventions (check all that apply) 7. Time Resusc Ended (Either "time of death" or "time left EC", whichever was 1st) 8. Patient outcome.	________ ________ ________ ❑ Too many urgent patient care issues to make time ❑ Did not feel it was needed. ❑ Other reason: ________ ❑ Respiratory ❑ Medical (includes seizure) ❑ Trauma ❑ Pulseless ❑ Intubation ❑ Defibrillation ❑ Code 3 Trauma Activation ❑ CPR ________ ❑ Alive ❑ Expired	1. Members Present ("X" box if present during debriefing) ❑ Chaplain ❑ Charge Nurse ❑ Child Life ❑ Family Advocate ❑ Pediatric Emerg Medicine Fellow ❑ Pharmacist ❑ Physician Team Leader ❑ Primary/ Documenting Nurse ❑ Resident ❑ Respiratory Therapist ❑ Secondary Nurse ❑ Other: ❑ Other: 2. Debriefing Physician. Team Leader Name: ________ 3. Debriefing Documenter Name (**NOT** same as #2 above; can be RN or Dr.) ________	1. Time Debriefing Started: ________ 2. What went well during our care for the patient? ________ ________ ________ ________ 2. What could have gone better during our care for the patient (ADD potential solutions if able)? ________ ________ ________ ________ 3. Was the Physician Team Leader (PTL) the **only** doctor calling out medication orders? YES NO 4. Was **anyone** confused at any time during the resuscitation about who was the PTL? YES NO 5. Time Debriefing Ended ________ 6. State: "If anyone wants counseling support, please see referral numbers at the bottom of this form"

DEBRIEFING FORM
FILL OUT LEFT SECTION BEFORE PATIENT LEAVES EC

Advice for Running A Team Debriefing

1. Pick a quiet or isolated space if possible—start by thanking members for being present & encouraging all members to participate.
2. State: "The purpose of debriefing is for education, quality improvement, & emotional processing; it is not a blaming session. Everyone's participation is welcome & encouraged."
3. State: "These debriefings usually take several minutes and if you have urgent issues to attend to, you are welcome to leave at any time."
4. State: "I will briefly review the patient's summary and then we as an entire team can discuss what went well and what could have gone better. Please feel free to ask any questions."
5. Proceed as team leader with a brief summary of the patient's course (<1 minute) and then proceed to the group discussion. Documenter (not team leader) records on this form.

*If anyone needs or requests referral for free counseling, call the appropriate institution at 832-824-3327 (TCH) or 713-500-3327 (BCM)

Updated 2/3/2012

Source: Reprinted with permission from Kessler, Cheng, and Mullan (2015).

Debriefings can also be useful in the emergency department setting. Exhibit 16.2 provides an example of a debriefing method known as DISCERN, or *debriefing in situ conversation in emergency room now.*

When combined, team briefings and debriefings significantly improve the perceived collaboration of OR personnel (Makary et al. 2007). While some may see the briefings as an interruption, most anesthesiologists, surgeons, OR nurses, and scrub technologists report that the benefits far outweigh any perceived inconvenience (Lingard et al. 2008).

CHAPTER 17

Simulation: The Low-Tech, Low-Cost Version

THE USE OF simulation in healthcare appears to be growing as more organizations embrace the approach to developing effective care procedures. Many institutions have built large simulation labs and equipped them with high-fidelity simulators and technology. While this infrastructure is helpful to any organization seeking to improve safety in care delivery, this chapter emphasizes how a hospital or health system of any size or margin can implement simulation without dedicating the lab space and purchasing the expensive equipment. Some simple steps can support an organization in building a low-fidelity, in situ simulation program.

SIMULATION IN HEALTHCARE

The Joint Commission considers high reliability in healthcare to reflect consistent excellence in quality and safety for every patient, every time (Loeb and Chassin 2013).

Why Simulation?

How does simulation support a high-reliability environment? Examples of the ways simulation can be used are presented according to

Weick and Sutcliffe's (2015) high-reliability principles, introduced in part I of this book: preoccupation with failure, reluctance to simplify, sensitivity to operations, commitment to resilience, and deference to expertise.

Simulation can be used in the context of the preoccupation with failure to build virtually fail-safe processes or procedures. Running simulations—experimenting with or testing and then measuring the outcomes of procedures—can identify weaknesses in the system prior to implementation.

Where sensitivity to operations and situational awareness (as discussed in chapter 15) are concerned, the organization can use simulation to identify issues that may occur with current inpatients, providing a real-time benefit to those patients.

Debriefing techniques can be considered a type of simulation in terms of commitment to resilience, whereby the organization conducts huddles following a difficult case or an environmental emergency. Staff are provided with opportunities for follow-up and resources, such as access to targeted employee assistance programs and critical incident stress management assistance. Debriefing also enables leadership to identify staff who may be at risk for burnout and provide a proper level of support.

Finally, in alignment with the principle of deference to expertise, once simulations have been run, feedback is gathered from the people who participated—those who do the work—about how to address system issues that have been identified.

Emerging research also supports the use of simulation in healthcare. Task training for competency and team building are two main areas of focus. In their article "The Top Patient Safety Strategies That Can Be Encouraged for Adoption Now" (Shekelle et al. 2013), the authors describe those patient safety interventions that are highly encouraged or encouraged on the basis of findings in the current literature. Those interventions that are highly encouraged include adopting bundles for addressing hospital-acquired conditions and using stringent hand-hygiene protocols. Use of simulation is an intervention that falls under the "encouraged" category.

History of Simulation in Healthcare

The history of simulation in healthcare can be considered in three main eras. First is the use of the so-called actual patient simulator. People might recall such a model from their initial CPR course using the mannequin Resusci-Annie. These courses were designed in the 1950s. Next, in the 1970s, simulation training was introduced for anesthesia residents and fellows. Then, in the 1990s, significant changes in medical education and a decrease in work-hour requirements led to the use of simulation to provide student physicians an adequate amount of clinical practice.

Now, a fourth era of simulation in healthcare is emerging as current patient safety efforts are driving its increased use in building teamwork and communication skills. The academic environment continues to create interprofessional simulation scenarios to enable physician, nursing, pharmacy, and respiratory care students to perform procedures as a team before they come together professionally following graduation.

SIMULATION FIDELITY

Simulation can be described in terms of a variety of types and levels of fidelity, or the degree of realism that can be produced during the simulation. In high-fidelity simulation, numerous components are joined to deliver the simulation experience. They may include task trainers for testing procedural competence; computer-based systems; gaming systems; actors posing as patients; and high-technology simulators modeled on humans that breathe, talk, and mimic other realistic elements. An example of high-fidelity simulation is the use of the entire care team and the equipment involved in cannulation for extracorporeal oxygenation, commonly known as heart–lung bypass.

Low-fidelity simulation may be seen as synonymous with low-tech, low-cost simulation. As described throughout the remainder of the chapter, it can be as simple as a tabletop walk-through of a scenario.

ORGANIZATION-WIDE SIMULATION ADOPTION

Healthcare continues to rely on traditional education and communication methods to disseminate new knowledge and its application. But policies, care pathways, and many other healthcare-related processes are increasingly lengthy and complex. Webinars, PowerPoint presentations, e-mails, and communication boards are not always adequate to build competency, whereas simulation can build not only individual proficiency but also team-based abilities. Latent system issues can be uncovered, especially with in situ simulation.

In short, simulation can bring the organization to a new level of safety and improve patient outcomes. It can be used throughout the organization for a variety of applications. From general team-based training to working with high-risk, low-volume procedures to practicing a move to a new geographic location to testing new processes or procedures, many healthcare activities are increasing their use of simulation.

Some particularly nontraditional uses for simulation include building competency skills for compassionate conversations, training for leadership responsibility, and building reliability in patient care handoffs. These and other areas are ideal for simulation because they assist educators in identifying human factors issues such as fatigue, ergonomics, distraction, stress, and resource and knowledge deficits.

Simulation is also much better than classroom or online teaching is at addressing what Sidney Dekker (2011) calls cognitive fixation. Cognitive fixation describes the phenomenon in healthcare where caregivers have a mind-set of "this and nothing else." In stressful situations, clinicians move along a decision-making path and may stay on that path even when symptoms emerge that should dictate different care decisions than those being made because of cognitive fixation. The other element of cognitive fixation is the thought that "everything is alright." Here, clinicians may believe that a patient is recovering in the face of threats to his or her well-being simply because one or two reassuring elements are present. Cases such as these are complex, and simulating them both proactively and following a real safety event can help build situational awareness. (Chapter 19 describes human factors in more detail.)

LOW-TECH, LOW-COST SIMULATION

To get started with a low-fidelity program of simulation, first, leaders should identify interested individuals who have had a positive simulation experience. Clinicians who have served in the military are often ideal candidates, as they are already well versed in the nature of simulation.

One approach to a low-tech simulation can proceed as follows: Find a unit nursing manager who is willing to try a just-in-time simulation on his or her unit. Then consider which patient scenarios could be developed into an interesting, teachable situation. Next, discuss with the manager what could potentially go wrong with that patient.

This straightforward process can be formalized as an exercise using the template in exhibit 17.1. The scenario template allows the leader to write up the scenario; designate the equipment that will be used; identify the supplies that will be needed; and provide an overview of the patient, including applicable patient vital signs and laboratory results. Other participants may be invited to join the simulation. As the simulation unfolds, changes to the patient's status can be tracked on the basis of the interventions recommended by the clinicians.

A simulation can be broken down into three steps: brief, execute, and debrief. The goal of the briefing is to build psychological safety. Start with introductions and a brief explanation of the roles involved in the simulation process. Emphasize that the goals of the simulation are to build communication skills and teamwork and to

Exhibit 17.1: Scenario Template

SCENARIO TEMPLATE
NAME OF SCENARIO

Scenario Objective:

Simulation equipment needed	Supplies needed

HISTORY FOR TEAM:

PATIENT VITALS:

TEAM SHOULD ASK FOR THE FOLLOWING:

LABS:

UPDATED ASSESSMENT:

START PROCEDURE:

END OF SCENARIO:

DEBRIEF:

assist in the discovery of system issues. Encourage the participants to ask any questions they may have and to act as they would in a real-world care scenario using the equipment and resources available to them. Also emphasize that what happens in the simulation stays in the simulation; no one will be reporting back to managers on individuals' performance.

Next, run the simulation. When you get to a logical finishing point, bring the team together to debrief. Steps for an effective debrief are as follows:

1. Offer a piece of positive feedback.
   - "That seemed to go very well overall."
2. Ask a participant to describe what occurred during the simulation.
   - "Can someone summarize the case?"
3. Engage the participants in an analysis of the simulation.
   - "What went well?"
   - "Where can we improve?"
4. Wrap up the simulation and thank the participants.
   - "Tell me one aspect of the simulation that you will take away from today's exercise."
   - "Thank you so much for participating. We know the experience can be uncomfortable, but this simulation will improve our patient outcomes."

Allow all simulation attendees to participate at an equal level. Make sure to assign accountability for follow-up on any system issues identified. In addition, consider whether these issues could be occurring in another department in the organization. Safety behaviors such as communicating clearly, asking questions, and speaking up can be identified during a debrief. Debriefing allows organizations to close the gap between current practices and high-reliability practices.

The best way to begin is to start where you are. Engage the organization's patient safety members to assist and give feedback; nursing and other department educators can also be helpful in this effort. Simulation does not have to be complex to be effective, and it can be a key process for hospitals and health systems concerned with becoming high-reliability organizations.

CHAPTER 18

Checklists[1]

CHECKLISTS ARE AMONG the most commonly used tools in high-reliability fields, such as aviation, the nuclear power industry, and the armed forces, to improve standardization, teamwork, and overall performance. In fact, in aviation, the use of checklists is mandatory; failure to follow the required checklist is a violation of flight protocol and considered a flight error (FAA 2017b).

USE OF CHECKLISTS IN HEALTHCARE

In healthcare, checklists have been used successfully in intensive care units (ICUs), emergency departments, surgery departments, and the anesthesia area. Early on, their use in healthcare was met with skepticism and resistance, and some clinicians continue to dismiss their utility. However, the results from applying the World Health Organization's (2009) *Guidelines for Safe Surgery* energized the concept of using checklists in surgery and anesthesiology. As a result, checklists are rapidly becoming established as the standard of care.

The WHO surgical safety guidelines are the best-known example of checklist use in healthcare. They were developed in response to findings that the most common location of adverse events in hospitals was the OR and that 43 percent of the incidents are considered preventable using current standards of care (De Vries et al.

2008). In fact, according to Weiser and colleagues (2008), "when published complication rates from surgery are extrapolated to a global population (estimated 234M operations performed annually), surgery may be responsible for 7 million complications and 1 million deaths every year."

Prior to the publication of those data, WHO launched the Safe Surgery Saves Lives (SSSL) initiative in 2006. The landmark study that emerged from that effort "provided evidence to support the introduction of the WHO Surgical Safety Checklist into surgical practice worldwide." The results reported in the study were compelling: Complication rates were reduced by more than one third and the number of deaths decreased by nearly 50 percent (Böhmer et al. 2012).

Two additional studies deserve mention that provide proof of checklists' efficacy. First, a study from the Netherlands examined a series of checklists known as the Surgical Patient Safety System, or SURPASS, which is applied to activities from admission to discharge (De Vries et al. 2010). The results were similar to the SSSL pilot study: The number of patients with one or more complications decreased from 15.4 percent to 10.6 percent, and in-hospital mortality decreased from 1.5 percent to 0.8 percent.

The second noteworthy study, by Neily and colleagues (2010), examined medical teamwork training, as well as the adoption of briefings, debriefings, and a surgical checklist, in 108 Veterans Administration hospitals over the course of 180,000 procedures performed. They found a 15 percent reduction in morbidity, significantly greater than in hospitals where this team training had not yet taken place.

HOW CHECKLISTS WORK

Checklists reduce errors, specifically errors of omission, by standardizing performance and reducing reliance on memory. As healthcare becomes more complex and as handoffs and shift work become more common, checklists are an ideal tool to combat errors. Not only do they improve team communication and situational awareness but they foster an improved safety culture as well.

CHECKLIST DESIGN

Healthcare has learned a great deal about checklist design from other industries. For instance, the Greenburg rule, generally associated with the airline industry, states that checklists should be no longer than one page. Further guidance from the airline industry advises teams to limit the number of items on a checklist to no more than nine, with five being ideal. Finally, checklist items should always be evidence based, and checklists should include items that prevent adverse outcomes. For example, checklists that are too long can slow the process of care, lead to unnecessary delays in surgical schedules, and alienate the users. Any of these issues may lead to the negative attitudes that defeat the purpose of a checklist.

One caution about checklists is that their frequent use can lead to "checklist fatigue," which itself may lead to errors if the checklists are seen as extraneous and unimportant (FAA 2017b).

EXAMPLES OF CHECKLIST USE IN HEALTHCARE

Checklists are used in many hospital areas beyond the ICU and surgical suites. They have become a critical tool for effective patient handoffs because they reduce technical and communication issues, not only for in-house handoffs but also with intrahospital transfers. They have also been adopted for use in radiology, labor and delivery, and endoscopy suites, to name just a few areas.

In the United Kingdom, the WHO checklist has been modified to include a team briefing at the start of surgery and a debriefing at the end (NPSA 2010), with more than 66 percent of the health trusts in England using the preoperative briefings. As of 2012, more than 4,000 hospitals in 122 countries have registered as users of the

WHO checklist, representing more than 90 percent of the world's population served by these organizations (WHO 2012).

Checklists in Emergency Situations

To address the use of checklists in high-stress emergency situations, Ziewacz and colleagues (2011) developed 12 "crisis checklists" for use during OR emergencies. They found that the use of the crisis checklists was associated with a sixfold improvement in adherence to critical steps.

The checklists cover emergency care for ten specific crises: air embolism, anaphylaxis, unstable bradycardia, unstable tachycardia, cardiac arrest with asystole, cardiac arrest with ventricular fibrillation, failed airway, fire (of the airway ventilation equipment), hemorrhage, and malignant hyperthermia. The last two checklists direct activity for two scenarios for which a diagnosis is unclear—hypotension and hypoxia.

CHECKLIST PROGRAM IMPLEMENTATION

Although the WHO checklist has been heralded as a major advance in medicine, the challenges to achieving widespread adoption have been significant. The most common of these continue to be negative physician and OR staff attitudes and a lack of buy-in or engagement. A 2011 article on engagement regarding checklist use in U.K. trusts found an astounding 77 percent of clinical staff failed to accept their use in practice (Health Foundation 2016).

The evidence from the Veterans Administration project mentioned earlier demonstrates that checklists are not a quick fix but rather require significant commitment at the grassroots level to ensure full and complete implementation. As is always the case in advancing change, education and local champions are the keys to success, and champions should have exceptional persuasion and negotiation skills.

No one who travels by air would reasonably object to the airline's captain and first officer using the preflight checklists prior to every flight. Our patients' surgical procedures should be treated no differently.

NOTE

1. Portions of this chapter are adapted from Walker, Reshamwalla, and Wilson (2012).

CHAPTER 19

Human Factors Engineering

IN ITS SIMPLEST form, human factors engineering is the study of how humans process information. This discipline takes into account such factors as physical environment, ergonomics, communication, distraction, lack of resources, stress, lack of awareness, fatigue, normalized deviance, and lack of knowledge (Gurses, Ozok, and Pronovost 2012). Taken one at a time, each factor can be addressed and overcome through awareness and training.

IMPORTANCE OF UNDERSTANDING HUMAN FACTORS ENGINEERING

In a complex system such as healthcare, at any given time one or more of these issues are likely at play, and when two or more of them interact, the chance of error increases. To understand how a particular error in healthcare delivery occurred, leaders must always consider the human factors involved. Comprehensive awareness of them allows staff and leaders alike to determine why people made the choices they did at the time because it sets the framework for valid cause analysis and subsequent interventions that lead to improvements in safety and reliability.

History and Examples of Human Factors

According to Meister (1999), the foundation of the science of ergonomics, a key human factor related to the physical environment, appears to have been laid in ancient Greece. A large body of evidence indicates that Greek civilization in the fifth century BC used ergonomic principles in the design of its tools, jobs, and workplaces.

Prior to World War I, the focus of aviation psychology was on the aviator. Wishing to enhance war pilots' performance in the air, researchers turned to studying the aircraft, in particular the design of controls and displays and the effects of altitude and other environmental factors on the pilot.

Also at this time, the field of aeromedical research emerged, triggering the need for testing and measurement methods. Studies on driver behavior gained momentum as Henry Ford began producing millions of automobiles (Meister 1999).

HUMAN FACTORS ENGINEERING IN HEALTHCARE

In healthcare, the adoption of human factors engineering approaches has been slow. Nonetheless, it is an essential aspect of achieving high reliability in care. Think of a busy ICU and consider some of the human factors listed earlier. The physical environment can be crowded and noisy. Often, clinicians and support staff need to hunt down supplies or equipment, causing distraction or increased fatigue. The unit may be understaffed, leading to stress. A patient handoff may be compromised by any number of issues, including communication issues, lack of resources, lack of knowledge, or fatigue. Normalized deviance may occur in the form of a work-around in the face of such factors. Lack of awareness, such as failing to grasp issues specific to a particular circumstance (situational awareness), may lead to faulty decision making. Lack of knowledge, which has been shown to increase the chances of committing an error by 30 to 60 percent, may lead clinicians and clinical support staff to make undesirable choices (Reason 1990).

HUMAN FACTORS SOLUTIONS FOR HEALTHCARE

Gurses, Ozok, and Pronovost (2012) offer suggestions for integrating human factors engineering into the healthcare space.

Education

A hospital or health system cannot fix problems it is not aware of. Because human factors engineering is not taught in the curricula of any clinical, ancillary, or healthcare management disciplines, the first step is to offer basic patient safety–oriented human factors training for hospital clinicians and administrators. Next, the organization should require healthcare professionals to participate in a project that applies the methods of human factors engineering, as many hospitals have already done in the areas of quality improvement, patient safety, and Lean techniques and strategies. People learn by doing. In the case of human factors engineering, staff and leaders might participate in a review of an error or incident that occurred in their department by walking through the incident with the help of the bedside staff. For example, to address a medication error that occurred from a pump programming issue, the review process could include setting up the pump at the bedside and walking through the entire process to demonstrate information about the error that could not be learned through discussing the event in a conference room.

Simulation

Chapter 17 discusses the value of in situ simulation. Simulation that takes place at the location where an error occurred—or is likely to occur—allows many human factors issues to be identified, not only with the physical environment but also with resources, communication, and levels of knowledge (Gurses, Ozok, and Pronovost 2012). One example is a multidisciplinary simulation for a respiratory condition. Team communication techniques, the equipment needed for the care of the respiratory patient, and processes to engage rapid response teams can all be included in the simulation scenario and then discussed in the debrief following the simulation.

Mistake Proofing

Next, Gurses, Ozok, and Pronovost (2012) highlight the importance of mistake proofing in healthcare. Though not called this at the time, mistake proofing began in 1853 with an elevator braking device developed by Otis Elevator Company. In a demonstration at the Crystal Palace Exposition of 1853 in New York, Elisha Otis rode an elevator above the crowd and had an assistant cut the cable. The elevator brake stopped the elevator—and Otis—from plummeting to the ground.

In the 1960s, Shigeo Shingo formalized mistake proofing as part of his contribution to the production system for Toyota Motor Company (Meister 1999). An example of mistake proofing in healthcare is the Broselow Pediatric Emergency Tape, used to reduce errors and increase the speed of treating pediatric trauma patients. The Broselow tape measure, which is color-coded according to height, is laid out next to the child, and the appropriate treatment color is determined. This color corresponds to an appropriately sized medical device and accurately dosed medications contained in packets of the same color, allowing the caregiver to begin treatment immediately without pausing to calculate dimensions and dosing measurements. In addition, dosages of commonly used medications are printed on the Broselow tape, further helping reduce errors (Grout 2007).

Mistake proofing is only effective if its tools are used every time an applicable situation arises. Organizations must be attuned to the activities taking place in patient care areas to ensure that clinicians and support staff are not taking shortcuts or using work-arounds in an effort to be more efficient. Ultimately, any perceived efficiency gains are eliminated when errors occur.

Forcing Functions

Forcing functions are another tool for addressing human factors. They are most frequently applied to equipment or supply designs that prevent the user from making a choice that could result in error. One example of a healthcare supply whose design incorporates a forcing function resulted from multiple instances of nurses administering IV fluids via feeding tubes and nutrients for feeding via IV tubes. As these instances continued to occur, healthcare tubing supply companies began to manufacture IV tubes that were incompatible with feeding equipment and feeding tubes that would not fit in IV pumps. In this way, nurses are "forced" to realize they have made an incorrect connection, thus preventing the error.

As with mistake proofing, forcing functions are in place to ensure safety, but they do not work if clinicians override them with their own techniques or procedures. Even forcing functions can be worked around if a clever nurse feels stressed and rushed.

As with other areas of the patient safety movement, healthcare delivery benefits from lessons learned in other industries in the field of human factors engineering and its integration into the environment. Human factors tools and methods need to be built into all aspects of patient care using education, simulation, mistake proofing, and forcing functions.

CHAPTER 20

Care Bundles

CARE BUNDLES ARE considered to be among the biggest success stories in healthcare safety. Many local, regional, national, and international projects and studies have demonstrated that care bundles are effective tools for advancing the implementation of evidence-based medicine; avoiding errors, including errors of omission; and improving patient outcomes.

WHAT ARE BUNDLES?

Horner and Bellamy (2012) define a care bundle as "a group of [evidence-based] interventions which when delivered together lead to a better outcome than performing interventions individually, representing an improvement over a non-structured approach." In other words, care bundles are sets of effective clinical interventions that are administered together to improve the standard of care and patient outcomes by promoting the consistent execution of the interventions. To be successful—that is, to improve outcomes to the greatest degree possible—all elements of a care bundle should be implemented in every appropriate patient 100 percent of the time. Anything less than 100 percent utilization is akin to having no bundle at all.

BRIEF HISTORY OF CARE BUNDLES

One early study of care bundles, by Berenholtz and colleagues (2002), used bundles to measure the level of quality delivered to patients by evaluating adherence to a list of interventions or treatments. In this manner, bundles were demonstrated to be a method for both measuring and improving the process of care.

WHY HEALTHCARE NEEDS BUNDLES

Since that time, a strong case has been established for the widespread implementation of care bundles in virtually every area of hospital care, from the ICU to the ED to the OR to labor and delivery to the medical–surgical floor. When bundles are implemented with 100 percent compliance, reductions in morbidity and mortality are significant (Council on Patient Safety in Women's Health Care 2015; Horner and Bellamy 2012; Surviving Sepsis Campaign 2015).

However, a well-documented finding indicates that the healthcare industry's overall adherence to evidence-based medicine is less than ideal. For example, intensive care patients often receive approximately half of the recommended clinical interventions—those that have been shown to significantly improve morbidity and mortality rates (Horner and Bellamy 2012). The failure of the US healthcare system to fully adopt bundles and other evidence-based care models must be overcome to move it forward on the journey to high reliability.

Benefits of Care Bundles

The benefits of bundles are many. They simplify decision making, help reduce errors in medical reasoning and errors of omission (forgetting to do something that is indicated), promote goal-oriented care, and help address areas of uncertainty or ambiguity by offering a practical, consistently applied solution for treatment. Additionally, care bundles are used to ensure the delivery of the minimum standard of evidence-based care. As suggested earlier, applying care standards based on evidence results in reduced complications, mortality, length of stay, and overall cost of care (Council on Patient Safety in Women's Health Care 2015; Horner and Bellamy 2012; Surviving Sepsis Campaign 2015).

COMMON TYPES OF CARE BUNDLES

Sepsis Care Bundle

The sepsis bundle developed by the Surviving Sepsis Campaign (2015) is the best-known example of a care bundle. Since its development in 2004, this bundle has been widely adopted internationally. It includes definitions, resuscitation guidelines, and ongoing management direction for severe sepsis and septic shock.

Levy and colleagues (2015) evaluated the effectiveness of the surviving-sepsis guidelines in an article published in *Critical Care Medicine*. With an aim to "determine the association between compliance with the Surviving Sepsis Campaign (SSC) . . . bundles and mortality," they measured compliance with the SSC resuscitation and management bundles by assessing the extent to which clinicians used the SSC guidelines in treating 29,470 patients (identified through the SSC database) from January 1, 2005, through June 30, 2012. Compliance was defined as evidence demonstrating that all bundle elements were used. The study included 218 community, academic, and tertiary care hospitals in the United States, South America, and Europe.

The authors found that increased compliance with sepsis care bundles was associated with a 25 percent relative risk reduction in mortality rate. In addition, for every 10 percent increase in compliance and every additional quarter-year of participation in the SSC initiative, a significant decrease was seen in the odds ratio for hospital mortality. Hospital and ICU length of stay also decreased by 4 percent for every 10 percent increase in compliance with the resuscitation bundle (Levy et al. 2015).

Central Line–Associated Blood Stream Infection Care Bundle

Another well-known care bundle was developed over a series of studies by Pronovost and colleagues (2006). It focuses on the prevention of central line–associated blood stream infections (CLABSI).

The economic burden of CLABSI on the US healthcare system is substantial. In one analysis, Horner and Bellamy (2012) estimate that each CLABSI occurrence independently increases length of hospitalization from 7 to 21 days and adds an attributable cost of about $37,000 (in 2002 dollars) per patient.

Elements of the CLABSI bundle include the following evidence-based recommendations from the Centers for Disease Control and Prevention (CDC 2017a):

- Guidance on handwashing
- Use of a full aseptic technique for central venous catheter insertion
- Use of a chlorhexidine solution for skin preparation prior to insertion
- Avoidance of the femoral site
- Removal of the line as soon as possible once it is no longer needed for care

Much of the evidence supporting these elements is based on small studies and observational data. However, adopting the combination of measures resulted in a dramatic reduction in infection rates per 1,000 catheter days from 2.7 to 0 within three months (Kirkland et al. 1999; Perencevich et al. 2003). Furthermore, in Michigan's statewide Keystone project, the mean rate of CLABSI dropped from 7.7 per 1,000 catheter days at baseline to 1.4 per 1,000 days after 16 months across participating sites (Stone, Braccia, and Larson 2005).

KEY ASPECTS OF CARE BUNDLES

What makes a good bundle? Following are some guidelines:

- Bundles generally include three to five evidence-based interventions.
- Each intervention should be evidence based or be widely accepted (signifying consensus) as good practice.
- Execution of the component bundle results in better patient outcomes than when the components are implemented individually.
- The bundle must be used for every appropriate patient 100 percent of the time.
- Each step, intervention, or treatment in the bundle should be auditable and able to be used to measure compliance with evidence-based practice.
- Compliance with the bundle is counted only when every intervention is completed or when the care team excludes a step for an acceptable, documented reason.

ADDITIONAL SUCCESS STORIES

Care bundles can be used to prevent a wide variety of clinical conditions. In addition to sepsis and CLABSI bundles, other well-documented bundles include those for ventilator-acquired pneumonia, catheter-associated urinary tract infections, pressure ulcers (PUs), and adverse drug events (ADEs).

For example, Nationwide Children's Hospital developed prevention bundles for PUs and ADEs (Brilli et al. 2013). Following adoption of the PU bundle, pressure ulcer rates decreased from a mean of 0.55 PUs per 1,000 patient days to a mean of 0.31 during 2012 ($p < 0.009$). Interventions included posting bundle compliance rates on units and directing units with low bundle compliance to create written action plans to address compliance gaps. As a result of these measures, PU prevention bundle compliance increased from 55 percent to 80 percent.

National Children's ADE prevention bundle was likewise successful, particularly when combined with post-ADE huddles or debriefings. ADEs per 1,000 dispensed doses decreased from 0.17 to 0.09 ($p < 0.001$) (Brilli et al. 2013).

Obstetric practitioners provide care prescribed by several perinatal bundles, including for the use of oxytocin in labor induction and augmentation, for perinatal monitoring, and for vacuum-assisted vaginal deliveries. The National Partnership for Maternal Safety has developed a four-phase bundle to treat obstetric hemorrhage (Council on Patient Safety in Women's Health Care 2015). The Safe Motherhood Initiative proposed a hypertension bundle that defines hypertension in pregnancy; specifies triggers to prompt further evaluation and treatment; and provides algorithms for common antihypertensive medication administration, checklists for eclampsia management, and educational materials for providers regarding quality improvement (ACOG District II 2017).

With all the evidence showing improvements in patient outcomes, including complications, mortality, costs, and length of stay, we can expect to see more bundles on the horizon.

CHAPTER 21

Shift Planning and Workload Management

HIGH-RELIABILITY ORGANIZATIONS KNOW the level of resources required to be successful. The most important of these is human resources. Until recently, healthcare has looked only at specific staffing levels in terms of the number of patients and the volume of procedures. More recently, hospitals and health systems have moved to base their staffing on patient acuity, staff knowledge, and staff capacity.

PATIENT ACUITY

Studies began to emerge in the literature about 15 years ago that lend support to the notion of *appropriate* staffing in healthcare—not just adequate patient-to-staff ratios—to reduce morbidity and mortality in a variety of patient populations. For example, Aiken and colleagues (2002) found that "in hospitals with high patient to nurse ratios, surgical patients experience higher risk adjusted 30 day mortality and failure to rescue rates."

More recently, Rogowski and colleagues (2013) studied the effects of staffing on infection rates in the neonatal ICU (NICU). They found that "understaffing is associated with an increased risk for [very-low-birthweight infant] nosocomial infection. Hospital administrators and NICU managers should assess their staffing decisions to devote needed nursing care to critically ill infants."

STAFF KNOWLEDGE AND EARLY WARNING SYSTEMS

While appropriate staffing might feel like common sense, shift planning and workload management in hospitals is complex. For instance, consider hospital staffing in areas other than nursing, where the majority of staffing studies are focused. Technology issues, such as failure or downtime related to electronic health records, IV pumps, cardiac monitors, and so on, rely on appropriate staffing in these departments to ensure that the equipment and systems can be fully utilized and patient care optimized, not compromised. If the environmental services department is not well resourced, patient care areas may not be at the highest level of cleanliness and infection rates may soar. Clinical professions, from nursing to respiratory therapy to rehabilitation services, now continually review their staffing practices in terms of patient acuity, assigned work hours, and workload. Refining these systems, and expanding them to nonclinical areas, enables the organization to identify increasing patient and customer needs and to appropriately resource all areas of the organization.

For example, hospitals have begun to adopt hospital early warning systems (HEWS) to identify when they are at risk of inadequate staffing from an organization-wide resourcing standpoint. Variations of HEWS, such as early warning scoring systems and modified early warning systems (MEWS), have been widely implemented across the United States. Developed in the United Kingdom, these scoring systems assist management in identifying high-risk patients who may deteriorate and subsequently trigger response by the rapid response teams. MEWS includes the following parameters: respiratory rate, heart rate, systolic blood pressure, consciousness level, temperature, and hourly urine output.

MEWS has itself been modified for pediatric patients as the pediatric early warning system (PEWS). PEWS does not monitor blood pressure or hourly urine outputs as parameters in the scoring; instead, it measures cardiovascular, behavioral, and respiratory parameters.

These warning systems are based on single-patient assessments. How do organizations assess for risk and respond appropriately when the whole organization is at capacity? Although the output of early warning systems does not indicate organization-wide trends, these systems can still offer guidance. Patient demographics and the size of and resourcing in the organization are also valuable indicators. In general, a HEWS score includes the percentage of occupied beds, percentage of staffing needs met, throughput data, and acuity level of current and scheduled patients. This score, or elements of it, is discussed at the organization's daily safety huddle or daily check-in (discussed at length in chapter 15). Staffing and recognition of upcoming safety concerns, including new and high-risk procedures, are part of the reporting structure of these huddles, which unit leaders attend. At the end of the meeting, they can discuss a plan for the organization in response to the elements of the HEWS that were highlighted.

Why is early recognition important? In high-reliability organizations, failure is not an option because lives are at stake. Industries recognized for high reliability, such as nuclear power and airlines, have shared numerous relevant lessons with healthcare, one of which is that they continually analyze the operational point at which safety declines, thereby having an awareness of how not to exceed the boundaries of safety. These boundaries are known in healthcare as boundaries of tolerable conditions of use (BTCUs) (Morath 2011). BTCUs are reached when a system moves toward unsafe practice as individuals gain the maximum benefit for the minimum perceived probability of harm.

Eventually, as errors and events begin to occur, management responds. However, contrary to the measures taken in the nuclear and airline industries, healthcare leaders tend to adjust by building an increasingly punitive environment characterized by more policies, additional process steps, and staff retraining—interventions that actually decrease safety in the organization. Work-arounds, normalized deviance, and decreased transparency become commonplace when an organization is not adequately resourced and has no mechanisms in place to identify increasing risks to patient safety.

CAPACITY

Meeting patients' needs is the first priority in healthcare, but recognition of organizational capacity is also important to prevent staff burnout and job dissatisfaction. Job dissatisfaction and burnout are highly correlated to high patient-to-nurse ratios (Garrett 2008). As discussed in greater detail in chapter 22, burnout symptoms can range from disengagement to anxiety and even lead to the individual leaving the profession.

Burnout and dissatisfaction both place patients at risk and result in staff turnover, which is costly to healthcare organizations. Thus, in high-reliability organizations, staff are highly trained, consistently mentally present, and very resilient.

Capacity is a relative term, and healthcare organizations need to define what it means in terms of their own safety boundaries. With that recognition, they must work toward resourcing their departments to address the community's need for and use of their services. Building a culture of safety to support this resourcing is imperative to becoming a high-reliability organization, and developing acuity systems; building in HEWSs; having low tolerance for situations in which acceptable conditions are barely met; and supporting staff through high-capacity, high-risk situations are all tools and tactics to exceed the goals of the organization.

CHAPTER 22

Emotional Safety for Employees

THREE DISTINCT DIMENSIONS of employee safety have been defined as personal, physical, and emotional. Personal safety relates to such issues as workplace violence, pedestrian safety, and emergency preparedness. Physical safety pertains to workplace injury and ergonomics. Emotional safety—often the last dimension healthcare organizations address, if they do so at all—includes the well-known phenomenon of burnout as well as the lesser-known issues surrounding the "second victim." First, this chapter discusses the second victim; later, it explores burnout and other emotional safety issues.

THE SECOND VICTIM

Effective support mechanisms for addressing the deeply personal and professional crises experienced by the second victims of medical error have not been widely implemented in the US healthcare system. The first victims, patients and families who experience harm, generally receive a well-coordinated and supportive response by a variety of professional groups throughout the organization. The second victim, the hospital staff member or physician who experiences an error, is often left to deal with the guilt and shame alone (Wu 2000). These caregivers and support staff can sustain deep and complex psychological harm, especially when the error results in a high degree of harm or death to the patient.

In the day-to-day operations of healthcare, loss and sorrow are part of the experience of being a healthcare professional. Feeling this loss as a result of systemic medical errors has been compared by some observers to post-traumatic stress disorder (PTSD). PTSD symptoms include sadness, fear, hypervigilance, disbelief, and shock, which can manifest in such physical symptoms as a rapid heartbeat, increased blood pressure, muscle tension, appetite disturbances, and difficulty concentrating. As with individuals suffering from PTSD, care professionals who experience a medical error often have concerns about how others view them, worry about losing their job or license, and dwell on the potential for involvement in litigation proceedings. They may find returning to work difficult and experience anxiety while at their job. These issues have the potential to put patients at risk.

The typical responses by healthcare workers, specifically clinicians, when they experience an error that leads to significant harm can be described in three categories. One is to leave their profession. This choice may be either voluntary or forced, as when the second victim's license to practice is revoked.

A second response is to remain in the profession in the same or a different institution. While this choice may signal to leaders and peers that the individual was not emotionally harmed by the event, without proper intervention, he or she may avoid certain situations or move to practice at a lower level of care and continue to experience PTSD symptoms or other physical or psychological problems.

The third course a professional may take following an error experience is to use the incident as a springboard to improve his or her practice and that of others. In a high-reliability organization with a strong culture of safety and transparency, these professionals are supported by having a forum in which to talk about their story and how it changed their practice. This opportunity allows the organization to highlight the use of safety behaviors and its organizational response to errors. Leaders of high-reliability organizations believe that, by allowing the second victim the chance to discuss the situation after it occurs, even though such discussion is painful and uncomfortable, the organization is building the safest professional workforce whose members become advocates for patient and employee safety and provide support for second victims (Grissinger 2014).

What is best practice in terms of responding to and supporting individuals who experience errors in healthcare? It begins with a strong culture of transparency (discussed at length in chapter 6). It is further supported by the creation of a supportive environment in which caregivers feel emotionally safe to disclose and take accountability for any event. When staff and physicians continually hear the message that errors are system based rather than the fault of individuals and see the organization respond to errors by correcting systemic gaps, they know that transparency is not about assigning blame. Furthermore, discussion of serious events at all levels of the organization enables staff to report these events and feel supported by the cause analysis process and then feel safe to seek further support if needed.

At the University of Missouri, MU Health System has developed a well-defined second victims program. Called forYOU, the initiative has been recognized nationally as a leader in the response to professionals in the wake of medical error events. As part of that program, the Three-Tiered Interventional Model of Second Victim Support, created by Susan D. Scott, RN, coordinator of patient safety at MU Health System, is employed. In the first tier, support is garnered from unit leadership (managers, supervisors, department chairs) and fellow team members. This group provides one-to-one support, the opportunity for discussion, and a professional collegial critique of the event. Tier 2 consists of trained peer support and makes available patient safety and risk management resources. This group is specifically trained in crisis management and provides one-to-one intervention, peer support and mentoring, team debriefings, and support throughout the cause analysis and any subsequent litigation. Staff who require tier 3 support are offered assistance through an expedited referral network including targeted access to an employee assistance program, a chaplain, a social worker, and a clinical psychologist. The expedited nature of this tier ensures that the individual receives prompt support and timely, ongoing monitoring (MU Health 2017).

Other organizations have developed incident rapid response teams. Similar to traditional rapid response teams, which rush to the aid of a patient in medical crisis, these teams are developed to respond immediately on behalf of the second victim when a serious event occurs. Teams are trained in critical incident management and consist of the chief medical officer or a designee, a patient safety specialist, and a hospital nursing supervisor or administrator. This makeup allows for both immediate feedback about the event and support from and connection to resources for the staff member.

BURNOUT AND RESILIENCE

For a healthcare institution to become a high-reliability organization, it must be able to support staff to prevent burnout and build resilience. According to the Lucian Leape Institute (2013) of the National Patient Safety Foundation, 33 percent of new nurses and 17 percent of new physicians leave their profession after the first year. One reason for these rates of professional separation is that only 37 percent of healthcare employers believe their employees are burned out. Both nursing and medicine can be characterized as having a survival-of-the-fittest mentality, limiting professionals' ability to recognize their burnout risk and request assistance.

Burnout symptoms can range from negative thoughts and worry to mental and physical exhaustion to anger, depression, and PTSD. These negative physical and emotional states lead to decreased feelings of well-being and ultimately impede a person's ability to provide safe, high-quality, and compassionate care.

How does an organization prevent burnout and build resilience in its workforce? First, the organization needs to admit that burnout exists and take into account times of high census and difficult cases and situations that can contribute to it. Leadership rounding promotes a sense of support and well-being, especially during stressful circumstances.

Next, leaders must encourage positive self-care for staff and recognize the need for true work–life balance. Another strategy is to offer organization-wide learning and support during and after difficult periods. Transparency about events, open discussions about support resources, and demonstrated recognition of stress build confidence that the organization cares about its team members. Finally, the building of meaningful relationships in departments, across organizational levels, and with patients and families can carry departments and individuals through ongoing stress.

Healthcare is built on brilliant and caring professionals and support staff who come to work every day with the purpose of helping people, not harming them. Healthcare leaders have a responsibility to build systems that support their workforce. A clinician should not have to leave his or her position after experiencing a system error or unaddressed burnout.

CHAPTER 23

Swarming: An Alternative to Root Cause Analysis

THIS BOOK HIGHLIGHTS numerous novel safety approaches that are not in widespread use in healthcare. Of particular interest are tools that solve or replace more cumbersome processes, especially those tools that are highly effective and relatively simple to implement.

Many clinicians and administrators have participated in root cause analysis and found the process to be complex and time consuming. RCAs often take weeks to complete and are sometimes perceived as punitive. But in 2009, University of Kentucky HealthCare (UKHC) quality and safety leaders developed a novel approach to RCAs, which they call swarming (Clements et al. 2014).

They were impressed by the successes of high-velocity organizations, such as NASA, and borrowed the concept of "swarm intelligence" from Bonabeau and Meyer (2001) and a similar idea from Spear (2008). Their version of a swarm is characterized as "a flurry of collective activity partaken by anyone and everyone available who is able to add value in the evaluation of an adverse event and development of possible solutions to prevent future occurrences" (Gartner 2010).

The UKHC swarm concept was refined over hundreds of episodes to its current iteration, which contains five key steps. Clements and colleagues (2014) describe the five steps as follows:

1. Introductory **explanation** of the process with description of the plan and the purpose, and reassurance of the participants that the SWARM will be conducted in a blame-free environment with legal protections to encourage candor.
2. **Introduction** of everyone in the room so there is familiarity combined with emphasis on respect by everyone—the group "attacks problems not people."
3. **Review** of the facts that prompted the SWARM.
4. **Discussion** of what happened, investigation of the underlying systems factors, and theorizing as to why and how it happened; that is, the RCA. This is more of a conversational forum, facilitated by someone well trained in safety science to ensure exploration of all the key issues. During this step, participants often rely on multiple tools to structure the conversation and clarify the problem, such as time line/flowcharts, Go-See, fishbone, Pareto, and 5 Whys. A time line, the single most important and consistently used tool in SWARMs, is an easily understood and simple tool to document the chronology of events. Through the use of a time line and repeatedly asking "how" and "why," problems and issues are more easily identified. The input of a heterogeneous group helps eliminate "confirmation bias" that may occur with a single person or a more homogeneous group. This focus on the interdisciplinary team attempting to understand the cause of an event soon after its occurrence is a strength of SWARMs.
5. **Conclusion**, with proposed **focus areas for action and assignment** of task leaders with specific deliverables and completion dates. After coming to a shared understanding of what happened and why, the team begins brainstorming fixes. Was this a staffing issue? Were there cultural issues such as poor communication or steep hierarchies? Does a process need to be

> standardized or simplified? Would a checklist help? Is there a feasible information technology solution? Though the interventions that involve "increased awareness" or "enhanced education" are important, the team attempts to propose solutions that change the process of care or build in forcing functions.
>
> The last 10 minutes of the hour are devoted to creating a formal action plan, and individuals are charged with completing any further investigation and implementing the action plan.
>
> A single participant is elected to act as the owner for this process and ensure that all other task leaders perform their duties as assigned and on schedule with a goal of completion within 60 calendar days. The weekly SWARM Closure Report . . . is shared broadly with system leaders to ensure transparency of responsibility of the person assigned to a task and timeliness to closure.

Swarms are scheduled for one hour. Participants include those directly involved in the event, a representative who has authority in and responsibility for the involved units or departments, medical and nursing leadership, and a senior hospital executive (e.g., chief medical officer, chief nursing officer, chief operating officer).

RESULTS OF THE SWARM APPROACH

As of 2014, UKHC had conducted more than 1,200 swarms. Approximately 75 percent of them were conducted within 16 days of the event. One example of an improvement from a swarm focused on preventing pressure ulcers during treatment with extracorporeal membrane oxygenation. The swarm led to a reduction in pressure ulcers from 5 of 11 patients (45.5 percent) in 2010 to 6 of 61 (9.8 percent) in 2013 (Clements et al. 2014).

PART V

COMMUNICATION

CHAPTER 24

No-Interruption Zones, or the Sterile Cockpit

HEALTHCARE BECOMES INCREASINGLY complex every year. Clinicians are expected to manage hundreds of pieces of information in their 8-, 10-, or 12-hour shifts. From alarms to equipment to family concerns to medical crises to care transitions and many more moving parts, new situations and technology challenge the most accomplished care provider.

No-interruption zones have been developed to address all these issues and allow clinicians to focus on the task at hand. Establishing these zones is among the easiest practice changes to introduce to the healthcare environment.

No-interruption zones are built on the aviation concept known as the sterile-cockpit rule. In 1981, the Federal Aviation Administration enacted the sterile-cockpit rule to help prevent errors and events that occur when a pilot's attention is diverted from his or her work. In 2011, distractions and interruptions resulting in omissions or inappropriate actions during flight operations accounted for 72 percent of the 76 reported airline incidents (NTSB 2014). The rule is composed of several regulations that prohibit crew members from performing nonessential duties or activities while the aircraft is involved in taxi, takeoff, landing, or any other flight operation conducted below 10,000 feet.

The sterile-cockpit regulation was prompted by numerous accidents that were found to be caused by pilot distraction and discussions about topics nonessential to the flight. One such incident was a landing error with Eastern Airlines Flight 212. According to the National Transportation Safety Board (NTSB), on September 11, 1974, Flight 212 landed 3.3 miles short of the runway at the Charlotte/Douglas International Airport in North Carolina. The NTSB determined that the probable cause of the incident, in which 73 people died, was "lack of altitude awareness at critical points of the descent due to poor cockpit discipline in that the crew did not follow prescribed protocols" (NTSB 1975). In the report, the time from initial descent to the accident's occurrence is documented in detail, revealing that the cockpit crew engaged in multiple nonoperational discussions while failing to acknowledge terrain warning alerts. Terrain warning alerts are designed to notify the pilots when the plane is within 1,000 feet of the ground. The NTSB reported that pilots tended to regard this alert as a nuisance, which appeared to be the case with the crew of Flight 212. No issues or malfunctions with the airplane equipment or the equipment at the airport were found.

Drawing parallels to incidents and events that occur in the hospital or healthcare setting is not difficult. For example, the lack of altitude awareness demonstrated by the pilots of Flight 212 mirrors failures in situational awareness in healthcare, as when alarm fatigue causes or exacerbates safety incidents in the intensive care unit (ICU).

If the just culture algorithm (explained in detail in chapter 31) were applied to the Flight 212 incident, the findings would reveal that no clear policies and protocols were in place at the time that would drive cockpit discipline. While discussion of behavioral discipline might have been part of initial education or orientation for the pilots, the absence of high-level protocols and periodical policy review likely resulted in normalized deviance: If the cockpit crew of Flight 212 regularly saw other pilots operating in a relaxed environment where nonoperational conversations were commonplace, the flight's pilots would have no reason to feel they were going against protocol. Similarly, the culture of piloting aircraft at the time perpetuated the idea that terrain warning alerts were a nuisance and thus not taken seriously.

High-reliability organizations avoid events and errors through communication, coordination, and accountability (Barnsteiner 2011). To become highly reliable in the complex environment of healthcare, organizations must have supportive processes in place to manage the wide breadth of information at hand. One example of such support is seen at Sentara Leigh Hospital in Norfolk, Virginia (Hines et al. 2008). The hospital uses a no-interruption zone at the medication dispensing machines, with a space surrounding each machine marked off by tape on the floor. Prior to designating the no-interruption space, these machines were areas where staff members would congregate and talk casually while one member was trying to dispense medications—some with complicated dosing requirements.

Now, when a nurse is in the taped area, it is considered a no-interruption zone where he or she may not be interrupted for any reason. Above the medication dispensing machines is a large sign with red print reading "No-Interruption Zone." In addition, the machines were relocated away from nursing stations and high-traffic areas. These innovations and the protocols surrounding them are taught during orientation, communicated to staff at meetings, and reinforced by supervisors in real time if a nurse is being interrupted while in the zone.

The use of no-interruption zones is supported by the Institute for Safe Medication Practices to prevent medication errors (Anthony et al. 2010).

Another use of no-interruption zones is during times of patient transitions. Nurse-to-nurse shift handoffs, the transportation of patients to the surgical suite or diagnostic areas, and the movement of patients from one nursing unit to another are all circumstances in which structured communication in an environment of little to no interruption supports a reliable handover. In line with the Lean framework, each patient transition that takes place should be conducted with the aid of a checklist that includes all pertinent patient information. It is in the communication of this information that the use of a no-interruption zone helps ensure clear, complete relays.

Concerns have been raised about engaging patients or families in these handovers because the presence of additional individuals who are not aware of the process may contribute to a chaotic environment. If this engagement is the norm, simple explanations at the beginning of the handover using a script, such as the one presented below, can convey the need for the no-interruption zone while inviting the patient's or family's participation:

> We use a no-interruption zone when we perform patient handovers. We want to make sure that we do not miss any information for your/your family member's care. Once we have completed our checklist, we welcome you to give us your thoughts and share any concerns.

While the use of no-interruption zones in healthcare is relatively new, they have yielded promising results already. A study in the critical care unit at Case University Hospital in Cleveland, Ohio, was among the first to report on the effectiveness of the no-interruption zones. In the three-week period following implementation, a significant decrease (40.9 percent) in interruptions had occurred (Anthony et al. 2010). Whether this decrease in interruptions is sustainable over time needs further investigation. However, given the amount and complexity of information and data that healthcare clinicians need to process and master, adopting no-interruption zones makes sense to lessen the chance of error. Human factors such as fatigue and lack of awareness can also be addressed through the use of these types of interventions.

CHAPTER 25

Intimidation: A Deadly Factor

INTIMIDATION IS PRESENT in every healthcare organization. Often, the perpetrators are unaware that they display this behavior. This chapter reviews the negative impact of intimidation, discusses current intimidation survey results, raises awareness of the issues related to intimidation, and presents strategies for removing intimidation from the healthcare environment.

In 2003, the Institute for Safe Medication Practices (ISMP) conducted a national survey to assess the presence of intimidation in healthcare. The results indicated that occurrences of disrespectful and disruptive behaviors interpreted as intimidation were not just isolated events but rather a cultural feature of healthcare work (ISMP 2004).

Ten years later, between July and August 2013, ISMP conducted a similar survey to determine whether and how intimidation levels had changed since the previous survey. The 2013 survey included 4,884 respondents—more than double the number of 2003 participants. Most were nurses (68 percent) or pharmacists (14 percent), but more than 200 physicians and almost 100 quality and risk management staff also participated in the survey. Of the respondents, 70 percent had more than ten years of experience. Highlights of the findings are described here.

The most frequent disrespectful behaviors reported were the following (ISMP 2013):

- Negative comments about colleagues (at least one incident was reported by 73 percent of respondents; 20 percent reported that they occurred often)
- Reluctance or refusal to answer questions or return calls (77 percent at least once; 13 percent often)
- Condescending language or demeaning comments (68 percent at least once; 15 percent often)
- Impatience with questions or hanging up the phone (69 percent at least once; 10 percent often)
- Reluctance to follow safety practices or work collaboratively (66 percent at least once; 13 percent often)

Although physical abuse (7 percent); throwing objects (18 percent); insults referencing race, religion, or appearance (24 percent); and shaming or humiliation (46 percent) were not encountered as frequently by most respondents, nearly a quarter reported that those behaviors were among the top three encountered during the previous year (ISMP 2013).

Why does intimidation continue to be an issue in healthcare? First, intimidating behavior is deeply rooted in the practice of healthcare delivery. From the beginning, healthcare has been defined by a hierarchy. Physicians were at the top of the ladder, followed by nurses, then support staff, and so on. The administrative side of healthcare was not much different, with the executives giving top-down directives to be followed in day-to-day operations.

As the patient safety movement gained strength in 2000 following publication of the IOM report *To Err Is Human*, this backdrop brought recognition of the depth and breadth of intimidation in the healthcare workplace. Safety culture surveys became commonplace, and executives started using them to gauge the level of hierarchy-based intimidation in their organizations. However, even with increased recognition, the deeply entrenched behaviors are difficult to eliminate.

Intimidation in the healthcare setting can be deadly. It may be as innocuous as a loud sigh or an eye roll or as overt as physical violence.

Regardless of the form, when a worker experiences intimidation, it can lead to reluctance to interact with the intimidating individual—or group of individuals, as with a specific discipline—even in the face of failing to meet a patient's needs. As is readily apparent, this reluctance or avoidance may lead to delays in or lack of care being administered. It may also lead to increased caregiver stress, which may result in errors.

Cross-departmental intimidation is also a concern, where territorial or other issues perpetuate dismissive or disrespectful behavior, causing increased communication and teamwork—again putting patients at risk.

Finally, intimidation in any form and at any level can lead to turnover. High turnover rates are not only financially costly but also result in environments filled with novice employees where real teamwork is never attained and institutional knowledge is reduced. Once again, these factors can place patient safety at risk.

An organization can address intimidation in several ways. The first is to craft a well-written code of conduct. Setting an expectation of respect, speaking up, and teamwork encourages these behaviors.

Second, executives need to be highly visible and demonstrably dedicated to patient safety and enforce this code of conduct. (Chapter 9 discusses the new roles for leaders in patient safety.) One of the most important ways leaders can address intimidation is to recognize the presence of an intimidation culture in their area of responsibility (ISMP 2013). To do so, they should encourage transparency in reporting disruptive behavior, regularly round to influence, and address any disrespectful or disruptive behavior they witness or verify as having occurred. Best practice is to confront intimidating behavior when it occurs or soon afterward. Furthermore, it should be done in a private discussion that the leader begins with a question so that the intimidating individual does not become immediately defensive. Questions such as, "Is something bothering you?" can start a discussion that reveals previously unknown reasons driving the behaviors. Just culture concepts (presented in chapter 31) may need to be applied, as the line between disruptive behavior and noncompliance to the code of conduct can be a fine one.

Finally, executives need to treat their peers and all staff and physicians with respect and openness to expect staff and physicians to do the same. To build this type of culture, Dr. Robert (Bob) Connors, president of Helen DeVos Children's Hospital in Grand Rapids, Michigan, implemented the "Call Me Bob" initiative in which he asked doctors to encourage staff to call them by their first name. This approach is discussed in more detail in chapter 29, but it bears mentioning here, as the goal is to make clinicians more approachable and to foster better communication on behalf of patients, resulting in reduced intimidation as a by-product (Ylisela 2015).

Peers can also support each other during a time of intimidation or a disruptive event. Encouraging peers to feel comfortable confronting intimidation is the key. Some hospitals have implemented a type of "code" response, naming it "code yellow," for example, which means someone in that area is having difficulty with another team member. Staff respond to the code by arriving at the location of the individual in need, as with a medical code, and help resolve the situation. If the situation cannot be resolved at the time of occurrence, the designated chain of command is instituted (exhibit 25.1). We often think of a chain of command in terms of clinical care, but in the case of an intimidation issue, a simple help chain can support staff and physicians during disruptive episodes. *Help chain* is another term for *chain of command* and conveys the idea that anyone can call for help either when he or she is not getting what is needed for patients or when practitioners or other staff are acting in an intimidating or disruptive manner.

Additional resources for addressing episodes of intimidation or disruptive behavior are the hospital's medical staff office and the system's human resources department. As mentioned earlier, the intimidating person may have no idea he or she is causing a problem. While that lack of awareness may seem puzzling to some, it is a symptom of not having been trained in a culture that openly and actively supports patient safety. Human resources or the medical

Exhibit 25.1: Chain of Command

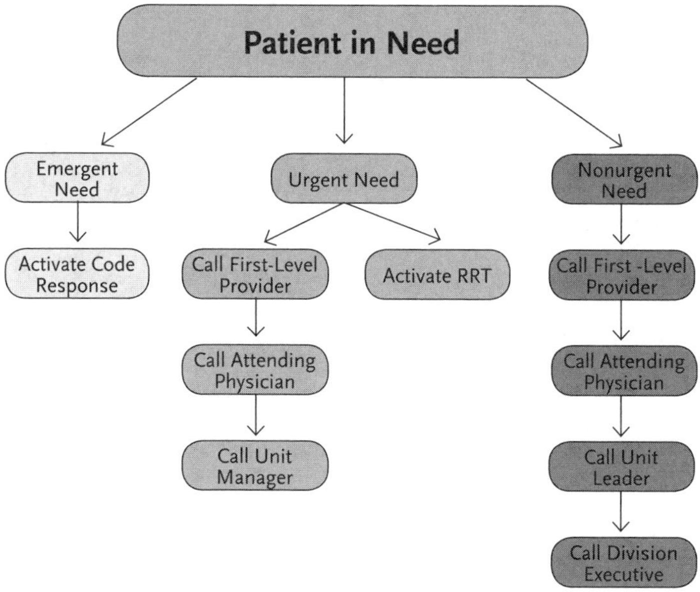

Patient in Need

- Emergent Need
  - Activate Code Response
- Urgent Need
  - Call First-Level Provider
    - Call Attending Physician
      - Call Unit Manager
  - Activate RRT
- Nonurgent Need
  - Call First -Level Provider
    - Call Attending Physician
      - Call Unit Leader
        - Call Division Executive

Note: RRT = rapid response team.

staff office can enable leaders to mentor and coach a person who is willing to change. This involvement sets the stage for them to help in the event that extreme behavior escalates to violence. In such a case, the consequences may include steps such as suspension and dismissal, which are guided by human resources or the medical staff office.

Intimidation in healthcare remains an issue. However, tools already in use in a culture of safety can be applied to lessen intimidation and disruptive behaviors. Taking action to eliminate intimidation can also save the career of someone who lacks self-awareness of these types of behaviors. Patients, staff, and physicians all benefit from active interventions in situations of intimidation and disruptive behavior.

CHAPTER 26

Standardizing and Structuring Communication

The greatest problem in communication is the illusion that it has been accomplished.

—Daniel W. Davenport

Communication is seemingly simple, but its execution is often ineffective, sometimes leading to tragic consequences. With "no less than 12.5 percent of verbal communication [being] misunderstood" (Nance 2012), communication failures were ranked as the second most common cause of sentinel events in the first six months of 2013 (Rodak 2013).

Following are some additional statistics that convey the impact of ineffective communication:

- An estimated 80 percent of serious medical errors involve miscommunication among caregivers during the transfer of patients (*Joint Commission Perspectives* 2012).

- Of the 901 sentinel events reported to The Joint Commission in 2012, communication was the third most common root cause of these events. Only human factors and leadership issues were more common causes (Rodak 2013).
- Research conducted from 1995 to 2005 demonstrated that ineffective team communication was the root cause of more than 65 percent of all medical errors that occurred during that period (Institute for Healthcare Communication 2011).
- Twelve percent of nurses do not speak up when witnessing an error about to be committed, even when they believe the potential for patient harm is high (Wachter 2012).

BARRIERS TO EFFECTIVE COMMUNICATION

Many factors influence the extent to which communications are effective. In general, differences in gender, culture, ethnicity, educational background, and communication style all can lead to communication failures. In the healthcare environment, an additional issue complicates the free flow of information: the existence of a hierarchical system among different groups as well as between senior and junior staff. These hierarchies are steep, and the authority gradients—the psychological distance between a supervisor and a subordinate—are huge, most commonly between the physicians and other clinical staff.

As Wachter (2012) states in *Understanding Patient Safety*, "All organizations need structure and hierarchies, lest there be chaos. Armies must have generals, large organizations must have CEOs, and children must have parents. This is not a bad thing, but taken to extremes, these hierarchies can become so rigid that frontline workers withhold critical information from leaders or reveal only the information they believe their leaders want to hear."

SOME SOLUTIONS

In other industries, and particularly in the military, communication is structured and standardized. This added structure aids understanding by ensuring clarity and reducing the ambiguity of the spoken word.

This discussion reviews solutions and tactics that can be used to overcome miscommunication and the hierarchy and authority gradients in healthcare institutions. It begins with straightforward tools and moves on to more complex solutions in subsequent chapters.

Repeat-Backs and Read-Backs

Many of us have seen movies set on submarines, where a captain's order is repeated down the line to ensure complete and exact understanding. Repeat-backs are an ideal tool for code blue situations where clarity and precise follow-through are critical. Following is an example:

Doctor: "Please give 0.3 cc's of 1:1000 epinephrine, IM, now."
Nurse: "Zero point three cc's of one to one thousand epinephrine, intramuscularly, now."
Doctor: "That is correct."
Nurse: "Giving 0.3 cc's of 1:1000 epinephrine, IM, now."

In this example, the physician is given the opportunity to correct any misunderstanding before a potent drug is administered.

Read-back is another technique to ensure that a sender's message is clearly understood by the recipient. This technique, in which the information is written down as received by the sender and then repeated back to the sender to ensure that no errors occurred in taking the message, has long been used in aviation. It has even been adopted for customer service or call-center scenarios, as when reading back a credit card number over the phone.

Read-back is a simple, effective, structured back-and-forth communication protocol that encourages clarification when needed, and it engages both communicators in the process regardless of the authority gradient between them. This commonsense approach to avoiding misunderstandings is an ideal way to receive and record laboratory values, radiology reports, and patient updates by phone.

Read-backs are used less frequently in healthcare than they should be. As Dayton and Henriksen (2007) state, "When other sectors of the economy have so convincingly incorporated read-back techniques in their operations to improve efficiency, safety, and customer satisfaction, ignorance of the role that read-backs can play in improving patient safety is difficult to justify." Encouraging all caregivers to use repeat-backs and read-backs in every situation where these approaches can potentially improve patient safety is a prudent measure.

Phonetics

The use of a phonetic alphabet, for example, saying Zulu, Tango, and Charlie instead of Z, T, and C, respectively, is not common in healthcare, but its use could mitigate communication errors.

Armed services personnel use a version of the military phonetic alphabet (an example of which, from the North Atlantic Treaty Organization, is shown in exhibit 26.1) to distinguish among letters because many sound similar when spoken over the phone or radio. For example, B, C, D, E, G, P, T, V, and Z all end with a long "E" sound. The correct letter can be difficult to identify when spoken quickly or over a poor connection. When communicating verbally in a stressful and noisy environment, such as the ICU, the difficulty is compounded.

As explained via Military.com (2017), "Clear, expedient communication is vital to any military operation, and the everyday method of conveying ideas isn't always suitable. Without a solid

Exhibit 26.1: Military Phonetic Alphabet

CHARACTER	TELEPHONY	PHONIC PRONUNCIATION
A	Alfa	(AL-fah)
B	Bravo	(BRAH-voh)
C	Charlie	(CHAR-lee) or (SHAR-lee)
D	Delta	(DELL-tah)
E	Echo	(ECK-oh)
F	Foxtrot	(FOKS-trot)
G	Golf	(GAULF)
H	Hotel	(hoh-TEL)
I	India	(IN-dee-ah)
J	Juliett	(JEW-lee-ETT)
K	Kilo	(KEY-loh)
L	Lima	(LEE-mah)
M	Mike	(MIKE)
N	November	(no-VEM-ber)
O	Oscar	(OSS-cah)
P	Papa	(PAH-pah)
Q	Quebec	(keh-BECK)
R	Romeo	(ROW-me-oh)
S	Sierra	(see-AIR-rah)
T	Tango	(TANG-go)
U	Uniform	(YOU-nee-form)or (OO-nee-form)
V	Victor	(VIK-tah)
W	Whiskey	(WISS-key)
X	Xray	(ECKS-ray)
Y	Yankee	(YANG-key)
Z	Zulu	(ZOO-loo)
1	One	(WUN)
2	Two	(TOO)
3	Three	(TREE)
4	Four	(FOW-ER)
5	Five	(FIFE)
6	Six	(SIX)
7	Seven	(SEV-en)
8	Eight	(AIT)
9	Nine	(NIN-er)
0	Zero	(ZEE-ro)

Source: Adapted from Navy BMR (2007).

understanding of what's being communicated, mistakes are likely to be made and may even be lethal." The same holds true in healthcare.

The point of the Military Phonetic Alphabet is not to obscure communications or speak in code but rather to communicate effectively by eliminating errors. Its use reduces the chance of misinterpreting verbal communication because each letter–word combination is unique such that it is unlikely to be confused with another letter.

This chapter covers the impact of poor communication; touches on hierarchy and authority gradients, which can hamper communication; and explores several simple yet highly effective communication tools: repeat-backs, read-backs, and phonetic alphabets. The next chapter reviews tools that help mitigate the authority gradients that hamper effective communication.

CHAPTER 27

Situation, Background, Assessment, and Recommendation Technique

THE JOINT COMMISSION notes that up to 60 percent of patient safety events feature some element of communication breakdown (Joint Commission Center for Transforming Healthcare 2014). Poor communication has also been identified as the primary factor in both medical malpractice claims and major patient safety violations, including errors resulting in patient death (Gregg 2013). The situation, background, assessment, and recommendation (SBAR) technique has been designated by The Joint Commission as an industry best practice for standardized communication in healthcare because it effortlessly structures critical information for spoken delivery.

SBAR accounts for the fact that the nursing and physician disciplines differ in their style of communication: Nurses are trained to report information in a descriptive, narrative fashion, while physicians are trained to seek or take note of only the key highlights in a patient's history. With SBAR, a high-quality communication includes the following elements:

- *The situation.* A description of what is occurring presently with the patient.
- *The background.* Discussion of the events leading to the patient's current state.

- *The assessment.* Objective information relayed by the informed clinician based on his or her assessment of the patient.
- *The recommendation.* The suggestion from the informed clinician to resolve the issue.

Each element should be communicated in two to three sentences at most.

SBAR is built on an evidence-based foundation and has been used in several other high-risk industries successfully, most notably in US Navy nuclear submarine operations and in the airline industry. Following investigation of numerous airline crashes in the 1970s, the primary cause was determined to be a breakdown in communication between the pilots in the cockpit. From that determination, the airline industry made a commitment to reduce airline accidents by developing a comprehensive safety program, and SBAR is one component of this program. As healthcare began to more carefully analyze its errors and events, industry observers found that communication errors added to many of the events and realized that a standardized communication tool could benefit clinicians (Blom et al. 2015).

Agreeing to adopt SBAR as a standardized communication tool is the first step in improving communication, but developing it as a habit without having a plan for implementation is difficult. Thus, education across departments and disciplines is necessary to launch an SBAR program. A generic approach to begin can be as simple as distributing SBAR-templated pads of paper to each nursing station phone, in nursing and physician break areas, and in areas where patient transitions occur. Stickers placed on telephones can remind staff to use SBAR. Individual departments may wish to consider developing SBAR templates that cover their most frequent communication elements.

SBAR IN CREW RESOURCE MANAGEMENT

The SBAR technique is a main component of the team-building practice adopted from the aviation industry known as crew resource management (CRM). As with other initiatives created for airline safety discussed in this book, CRM was developed in response to critical and fatal errors committed by flight teams. The method has since been adopted in the healthcare industry to build communication, cooperation, and information sharing.

The overall goal of CRM is to diminish the human factors that can cause error. Concerned with cognitive and interpersonal skills rather than technical knowledge, CRM attempts to optimize the use of available resources, such as equipment, procedures, and people, to promote safety and enhance efficiency.

Support for the implementation of CRM in healthcare is extensive. The Agency for Healthcare Research and Quality, the Institute for Healthcare Improvement, The Joint Commission, and the National Quality Forum all suggest the use of CRM to address communication and teamwork issues. However, widespread implementation of CRM has been slow. An organization that is interested in improving safety outcomes might first implement SBAR as a communication tool and then add CRM.

Although education corporations and other companies offer courses in CRM, organizations may improve teamwork outcomes by using just-in-time, in situ simulation to address communication and interpersonal relationship dynamics. Before commencing, communication and teamwork goals should be determined, with the understanding that all participants have an equal voice in selecting them. During these simulations, leaders must be sure to include the organization's safety specialist to assist in facilitating the briefing and debriefing process. As part of the debriefing, skills such as speaking up, asking clarifying questions, and using the SBAR technique can be prioritized. (Review chapter 17 for information on implementing a low-fidelity in situ simulation program.)

Errors and incidents that arise from communication and teamwork issues are often complex and require a multifaceted approach to resolve. SBAR is a communication method that can be implemented over time to focus attention on the details that influence the opportunity for error. CRM is a teamwork-based system that can build on SBAR and further decrease communication errors and events. The use of simulation is a best practice for fully incorporating SBAR and other teamwork elements of CRM.

CHAPTER 28

Tools for Acquiring the Skill of Assertiveness

A NURSE OBSERVES a physician not washing her hands before examining a patient. A radiology technician sees a spot on an X-ray that seems concerning, but the radiologist reading the X-ray states that it is normal. An environmental services worker watches as a nurse technician haphazardly cleans a room and then reports that it is ready for the next patient.

Ideally in each of these situations, the team member who observes the error feels free and safe to speak up about it. That is not always the case. The entrenched hierarchy in healthcare and persistent intimidation among healthcare workers (described at length in chapter 25) can impede the ability of smart, highly competent, and well-meaning staff and physicians to do the right thing.

Tools have been designed to assist healthcare workers in speaking up when they may not feel comfortable doing so, including:

- the CUS communication strategy, where CUS represents *concerned*, *uncomfortable*, and *safety issue*, and
- ARCC, which stands for the phrase *Ask* a question, make a *request*, voice a *concern*, and use the *chain of command*.

THE NEED FOR COMMUNICATION ASSERTIVENESS TOOLS

Are tools necessary to encourage healthcare workers to speak up? According to an Institute of Safe Medication Practices survey on workplace intimidation, 17 percent of respondents felt pressured to accept a medication order despite concerns about its safety on at least three occasions in the previous year; 13 percent had refrained from contacting a specific prescriber to clarify the safety of an order on at least ten occasions; and 7 percent said that in the previous year, they had been involved in a medication error where intimidation played a part (ISMP 2004). Specific to nurse-to-nurse intimidation, a study conducted at St. Joseph's University in Philadelphia explored the components, characteristics, consequences, and effects of abuse to understand the dynamics of verbal abuse of nurses in the workplace. More than a quarter of respondents (27 percent) reported that the most frequent source of abuse was other nurses (Rowe and Sherlock 2005).

Healthcare workers, as with most other human beings, will do what is necessary to avoid painful interactions. They may feel their patient is not getting the care or treatment he or she needs but delay calling a caregiver because they have had a previous negative interaction with that individual. A nurse may avoid alerting another caregiver if she is worried that she will be shamed, put down, or made to feel stupid.

CONCERNED–UNCOMFORTABLE–SAFETY ISSUE

CUS is a play on words to assist healthcare workers to remember to speak up when they are concerned, are uncomfortable, and feel a patient safety issue is present. CUS was formed as part of the TeamStepps program to improve teamwork and communication among healthcare workers (AHRQ 2014). In this strategy, workers are encouraged to use these terms to highlight the concern they have about a patient or situation so the listener engages more actively in the conversation.

Another way to heighten this awareness is to state a safety phrase, such as "I have a concern," that is built into the organization's lexicon as a standard way of communicating. This phrase, much like the CUS methodology, represents a red flag that says to anyone in the organization that the speaker feels the patient is at risk and the listener needs to attend carefully to the extent of the concern.

ASK–REQUEST–CONCERN–CHAIN OF COMMAND

The ARCC tool is an assertion and escalation technique. This stepwise approach enables staff and physicians at any level of the organization to begin a safety dialogue with a light touch to voice their concern and escalate the tone as necessary up to the engagement of leadership when they feel a patient's needs are not being met or risky behavior is taking place. Revisiting the hand-washing example at the start of this chapter, the nurse's use of ARCC could transpire as follows:

- *Ask a question*—"Dr. X, did you miss an opportunity to wash your hands?"
- *Make a request*—"I have the hand sanitizer here. Please use it before you get started."
- *Voice a concern*—"I have a concern that if you don't wash your hands, the patient will be at risk for infection."
- *Use the chain of command*—With discussion points exhausted, the nurse has the option of calling the next up in command, such as a charge nurse or the nursing supervisor or manager, to speak with the physician or initiate a follow-up interaction. Some institutions have physician executive call schedules in place for just-in-time

discussions of physician concerns or behavioral issues that put patients at risk.

Leadership must support the use of the CUS words and ARCC. If staff do their part and speak up but go unsupported in doing so, they will not continue to speak up. This choice may leave a patient at risk.

Especially in cases where the chain of command is leveraged, the onus is on novice staff members to muster the courage to use the chain of command. In turn, the response from leaders must be to thank the staff member, resolve the issue, and update the staff member as to the resolution of the concern. Leadership can also support staff on an ongoing basis by discussing the use of these strategies and tools at staff meetings and through other modes of communication.

CHAPTER 29

First Names Only

THIS CHAPTER TAKES an in-depth look at hierarchy and authority gradients and the lessons learned in other industries that can be adopted in healthcare.

In today's airline industry, the cockpit crew—the captain and first officer—refers to each other by *first names only* on flights. This protocol ended the practice of the 1970s and earlier whereby junior pilots addressed their senior counterparts as "Captain," "Sir," or "Ma'am."

This change was deliberately adopted to flatten the inherent hierarchy and shrink the authority gradient between junior and senior officers. It is meant to encourage a junior first officer to speak up to or ask a question of more senior colleagues, with the aim to abolish the perception that speaking up is equivalent to challenging the captain's authority.

As noted by Lawton and Armitage (2012; emphasis in original), "During announcements, pilots often introduce themselves to passengers using their titles and surnames; and they wear uniforms that visibly signify their status and rank. But in the cockpit, formal titles are used only in extreme circumstances to draw attention to the gravity of a situation, such as when a co-pilot follows the *PACE protocol* to challenge the performance or behavior of a captain."

However, in healthcare, nurses, students, and residents are still expected to refer to established physicians by their title and last name, for instance, "Dr. Byrnes" rather than "John." Use of formal titles reinforces the hierarchy in medicine and can create significant communication barriers among team members, prevent critical feedback from being delivered, and be a major contributor to medical errors.

Clearly, this issue is not straightforward (see sidebar on this page). Nevertheless, if staff address each other using only first names, patient safety might improve if the practice promotes a culture in which even the most junior team members are comfortable speaking up whenever they perceive a hazard to patient welfare.

A HEALTHCARE CASE STUDY

Helen DeVos Children's Hospital (HDVCH) in Grand Rapids, Michigan, was an early adopter of high-reliability tools and processes. In fact, the organization saw a 90 percent drop in serious safety event rates. It has achieved high marks in clinical quality and

Discomfort with First Names Only

For years, I have asked my nursing colleagues to call me John, and most of the time, they gladly accommodate my request. But over the years a few have felt uncomfortable addressing me without using the doctor title. One of my most esteemed colleagues, a nurse who is a major in the US Air Force, simply will not make the shift. We have talked about it monthly for almost half a year, and I have as yet been unsuccessful in convincing her to call me John. She stands firm in her perspective that it would be "disrespectful to you and all the hard work you've done to earn it, to call you anything other than Dr. Byrnes."

I certainly appreciate and respect her sentiment. That said, I feel the use of "Dr. Byrnes" inserts an air of strict formality into our professional relationship, and with it, the hierarchy remains.

—J.B.

patient safety, and its president, Bob Connors, MD, was recognized by the National Patient Safety Foundation for his leadership in improving patient safety.

However, despite the high-functioning teams and overall organizational success in quality and patient safety, Connors felt HDVCH still faced some barriers. He was unhappy with the lack of progress on annual safety culture survey scores and questioned staff members' ability to speak up when they had concerns about patient care. He felt that change was needed to overcome the traditional medical culture that still thrived to the point that physicians were contributing to safety issues by perpetuating the hierarchy in medicine, and some by exhibiting intimidating behaviors. Authority gradients remained as well.

So, he launched a new initiative, the Call Me Bob campaign. Using himself as the leading example, Connors asked all staff to call him by his first name. The gesture had the intended effect of starting conversations across the organization.

Furthermore, Connors asked everyone in the organization to adopt the first-name-only approach when interacting with each other. He engineered an extensive communication campaign and even changed the organization's employee badges—including those of physicians—so they highlighted everyone's first name. He personally led the campaign and held individual conversations with many staff and physicians about the initiative.

The operating room staff were early adopters, with the nurses and most of the surgeons immediately jumping on board with the concept. Curiously, most of the holdouts were anesthesiologists. But Connors never gave up, and they were eventually won over as well.

The Call Me Bob campaign appears to have strengthened relationships, the authority gradients are disappearing, and an ease of interaction is being observed between clinical staff and physicians (Connors 2017).

The use of first names only carries a "shock factor" when first mentioned in the formal environment of healthcare, but if it is deemed acceptable and appropriate for the airline industry, it seems more than reasonable for healthcare.

PART VI

GUIDELINES

CHAPTER 30

Red Rules[1]

As healthcare works to create a culture of safety, many organizations are adopting safety practices from highly reliable organizations (HROs) in other industries. One safety practice used by aviation, manufacturing, and the nuclear power industry—red rules—has sparked interest in healthcare. This chapter reviews how red rules are intended to work, discusses the benefits of red rules, and offers examples of their success in healthcare organizations.

WHAT ARE RED RULES?

Red rules were developed by E. C. Simpson, a retired nuclear industry executive (Jones and O'Connor 2016). In healthcare, red rules are applied to reduce the number of incidents of harm to patients. One of the most common healthcare red rules is the requirement to take a time-out, or pause to complete the surgical checklist, prior to a surgical procedure. The use of time-outs should be reserved for activities that carry the highest level of risk to patients, or staff, if not performed exactly as intended each time.

Some of the most common red rules found in healthcare include the following:

1. Verify the identity of patients using two forms of identification.
2. Label all specimens at the patient's bedside immediately after gathering them.
3. Use sterile surgical instruments in surgery.
4. Wear masks, gowns, and sterile gloves during a surgical procedure.

At their most basic, red rules are rules that cannot be broken, as with the long-held practice of a sterile surgical environment dictated by red rules 3 and 4 in the list above. They are few in number, easy to remember, and used for processes that can cause serious harm to patients and, in some cases, to caregivers.

Red rules are designed to be followed exactly as specified in all but the most urgent situations. Furthermore, every caregiver is expected to "stop the line"—a phrase taken from the assembly line in manufacturing whereby any worker is authorized and, in fact, obligated to halt the movement of the line when an error occurs or a defect is found—if a red rule is violated. Red rules are intended to give every worker the ability to speak up and stop a care process when the rule is not being followed. In addition, management is expected to support the stoppage when the rule is violated, regardless of the financial impact or disruption to those involved.

Examples of Common Red Rules in Everyday Life

In most US workplaces, a few rules are expected to be followed that stem from well-established societal norms—they are understood by almost everyone and intended "to [never] be broken under any circumstance by anybody in the organization" (ISMP 2008). Examples include the strict prohibition of sexual harassment and of working under the influence of drugs or alcohol.

The April 24, 2008, issue of *ISMP Medication Safety Alert* provides the following example of a red rule used in everyday life:

> The use of seatbelts could be an example of a red rule that everyone should follow. If an individual is not "buckled up" when the automobile pulls out, any driver or passenger in the car—child, spouse, friend—should be empowered to speak up, tell the individual who is not wearing his seatbelt to buckle up, and cause the vehicle to stop until the action is completed.

CONFUSING RED RULES WITH POLICIES AND PROCEDURES

An important issue regarding red rules is to avoid confusion between red rules and organizational policies and procedures (Scharf 2007). Think of policy and procedure compliance as always expected but with allowance to violate a policy or procedure if circumstances warrant, as when staff are not able to follow the rule or when violating the rule is the best course of action. The following Institute for Safe Medical Practices (ISMP 2008) safety alert provides an example:

> [I]n an environment where bar-coding technology is available, policies and procedures that call for practitioners to scan all medications before dispensing or administering them would certainly be considered crucial. However, circumstances will arise when scanning is not possible due to technology glitches, product idiosyncrasies, or emergency situations. Thus, compliance with bar-coding technology cannot be considered a red rule unless the organization has processes in place to ensure that not scanning a medication is a very rare event, and anyone can "stop the line" when it doesn't occur.

TOO MANY RED RULES ARE DANGEROUS

Reliance on too many red rules can lead to rule-dependent behavior that suppresses the use of critical thinking skills. Furthermore, too many red rules are difficult to remember and follow at all times. Organizations must monitor the number and appropriateness of red rules, keeping their application to a minimum and ensuring that they are used in situations for which they yield the optimal outcome.

RED RULE DESIGN GUIDELINES

In differentiating between red rules and an organization's policies and procedures, the following guidelines should be kept in mind:

- Red rules are designed to be followed every time, without exception.
- When a red rule is violated, anyone, from frontline staff to physicians to nurses to managers, has the authority and responsibility to stop the line. In other words, the process of care is stopped to protect the patient or employee from harm.
- Leaders always support the work stoppage.
- The problem that triggered the red rule is immediately addressed. For instance, if a ventilator is not plugged into a red emergency outlet, the situation is immediately corrected.

RECOMMENDED PROCESS FOR RED RULE DEVELOPMENT

To help ensure success in the development of and adherence to red rules, first, an interdisciplinary team, including representation from senior leadership and medical and nursing staff, should be formed.

Its main purpose is to carefully consider each suggested rule to make sure it meets the criteria in the earlier list of guidelines.

Second, extensive communication and training must be provided to all relevant staff and repeated at regular intervals to ensure that all staff and physicians clearly understand the need for the red rule, how the rule is used, how breaches are handled, and how the rule contributes to the organization's overall patient safety efforts.

Third, an audit process should be in place to measure compliance with the red rule, especially in the early days of rollout and implementation. Once the rule is hardwired into the organization's standard work processes, the determination and dissemination of exceptions to the rules are likely all that will be needed to ensure success.

ONE MORE HEALTHCARE RED RULE

This section discusses in detail another common red rule in healthcare: conducting sponge and instrument count reconciliation in surgery.

Reconciliation of Sponge and Instrument Counts in Surgery

Toward the end of a surgical procedure, reconciling the sponge and instrument count—that is, counting the numbers of sponges and instruments to make sure they match the presurgery numbers—before closure of an incision is considered standard practice. The process is a good example of a red rule and the primary safety practice to prevent the retention of foreign objects inside the patient after surgery.

If the surgeon attempts to close the incision before reconciliation is completed—a breach of the red rule—anyone in the room is permitted, and encouraged, to halt the process until the reconciliation process has been conducted and the correct numbers achieved.

If a breach does occur, physician and administrative leaders must hold the physician accountable for his or her actions, determine the reasons for the breach, and fully support staff who attempted to stop the process.

Even though this red rule is an established practice in all operating rooms across the country and supported by national healthcare regulations, incidents of foreign object retention following surgery continue to occur. The reasons are numerous and beyond the scope of this chapter. Suffice to say here that red rules have a definite place in healthcare. Remembering the medication error that killed my grandfather, a red rule that protected the medication administration process would likely have saved his life. Such a red rule might read as follows: "When nurses are working with or administering medications, they are *not* to be interrupted." This red rule creates a no-interruption zone, and it might have spared my grandfather's life.

NOTE

1. Portions of this chapter were adapted from ISMP (2008).

CHAPTER 31

Just Culture: Akin to a Whack-a-Mole Game

In the buildup to high reliability, the effectiveness of leadership resides in leaders' willingness to support a culture of transparency that allows the collection and analysis of all data related to adverse events and near misses (Dekker 2007). For this shift to occur, leadership must respond to these events in a fair and systematic matter.

PATIENT SAFETY AND THE NO-BLAME CULTURE

While historically healthcare has been known to operate under a big-stick disciplinary process, more recently, healthcare providers have integrated a no-blame culture. The advent of the no-blame culture was seen as a revitalizing change in a healthcare system that was marred by punitive disciplinary systems and overshadowed by the litigious landscape.

Limitations of Systems Thinking

Rather than the solution to safety issues in healthcare, however, the no-blame culture is now seen as enabling those who may put patients at risk. In the wake of healthcare's maturation in patient safety efforts, some observers believe a balance is needed that weighs learning from errors and events against managing performance violations. The idea that emerged from the no-blame mind-set, that all errors are a result of systemic issues, enables leaders to avoid holding difficult conversations with individual staff members who may be putting patients at risk. Some leaders prefer to "go along to get along," ignoring instances of staff noncompliance with safety rules. But a unit leader who witnesses a staff member failing to act in accordance with rules, protocols, or expectations and avoids correcting that behavior invites others to ignore the rules, with the ultimate result that patients are harmed.

One aspect of systems thinking is known as the noncompliance equation, described by Healthcare Performance Improvement (2009) as a combination of coworker coaching, perceived burden, and perceived risk. The equation dictates that these elements be considered to determine whether an error meets the criteria of a systems issue. First, in terms of coworker coaching, the question to ask to achieve peer-to-peer understanding is, "Would another professional in the same situation experience the same error?"

Second, to address the perceived burden component of the equation, a leader is designated to ask, "How difficult is this process to perform?" This consideration includes the number of work steps, the availability of needed resources—human and other—the complexity of the process, time pressures in play at the time of the error, and the nature of the environment in which it occurred.

Third is the question of perceived risk. As with the second element of the noncompliance equation, a leader is tasked to ask the key question: "Do our staff and/or physicians recognize the risks of performing this process or procedure?" Here, the act of recognition is tied to the perception of risk, an area in which the same characteristics that make a clinician excel can lead to his or her failure to protect a patient's safety. Sometimes, highly skilled clinicians who are capable of performing the most complex tasks complete them without having to apply their critical thinking skills. They are not always mindful of what could go wrong in the process or procedure; their competence drives noncompliance in the form of a work-around.

THE SOLUTION TO A NO-BLAME CULTURE

Historically, the US healthcare system has tended to hold physicians accountable only for those transgressions that are related to regulatory or administrative standards set by their own professional organizations, such as the American Medical Association or The Joint Commission. Barriers that prevent hospitals and health systems from holding physicians accountable to patient safety standards include weak medical staff systems, ineffective policies, and fluid structures. In these cases, physician peers serve as the reviewers, and they tend to put themselves in the shoes of the physician being reviewed. Not wanting to "get them in trouble," these peer reviewers may skirt the accountability issue and refer to the errors committed as *known complications*. In short, policies may be written to hold physicians accountable, but those policies may not be applied.

The just culture concept serves as an antidote to issues of patient safety accountability because it allows leaders to not only question the clinician about what happened in the commission of an error but track and trend individual and group performance.

What Is Just Culture?

The term *just culture* derives from David Marx's (2001) description of the so-called four evils: human error, reckless conduct, negligent conduct, and knowing violations. A just culture enables leaders to overcome these evils in their organization by deciding where and when to assign individual culpability when an error occurs. The just culture or performance management algorithms are designed to give leaders a step-by-step approach to performing cause analysis and responding to the staff and physicians who are involved in an error. Furthermore, Marx's description of the four evils includes recommended follow-up actions for directing consistent responses to those individuals.

Types of Errors

Three types of errors and responses are outlined in the just culture algorithms. The first type of error is the result of reckless or deliberate harm, as when a person acts with conscious disregard for the substantial risk present to the patient or in the environment. To address this error type, the first question a leader asks is, "Did this person act with malicious intent?" If the answer is yes, the leader needs to involve the human resources department as soon as possible to respond according to the organization's established protocol. A criminal component may be present in this type of situation, so the legal department may also become involved. While these types of errors occur least frequently, they must be considered as part of an investigation.

The second type of error is the result of negligent conduct or at-risk behavior, as when the person has not taken the appropriate steps to achieve an expected positive outcome. In this case, leadership needs to ask whether a system component is at play in the commission of the error. The noncompliance equation applies in this type of error, as leaders must determine whether the organization has made it easy for the person to do the right thing. The next question is, "Does the individual understand the risk inherent in his or her behavior?"

Leaders may also apply a substitution test by asking whether a similar person placed in that situation would have experienced the same error. If the leaders determine that the error was caused by a system issue, they need to update their processes. If they conclude that the system is easy to manage and the person does understand the risk, coaching should take place following the error. Regardless of whether the error is systemic in nature or the result of negligent

Exhibit 31.1: Incident Decision Tree

Start here

Deliberate Harm Test

Were the actions as intended?
- YES → Were adverse consequences intended?
  - YES → Consult NCCA or relevant regulatory body. Advise individual to consult Trade Union Representative. Consider • Suspension • Referral to police and disciplinary/regulatory body • Occupational Health referral. **Highlight any System Failures identified**
  - NO → Incapacity Test
- NO → Incapacity Test

Incapacity Test

Does there appear to be evidence of ill health or substance abuse?
- YES → Does the individual have a known medical condition?
  - YES → Is there evidence that the individual took an unacceptable risk?
  - NO → Consult NCCA or relevant regulatory body. Advise individual to consult Trade Union Representative. Consider • Occupational Health Referral • Reasonable adjustment to duties • Sick leave. **Highlight any System Failures identified**
- NO → Foresight Test

Foresight Test

Did the individual depart from agreed protocols or safe procedures?
- YES → Were the protocols and safe procedures available, workable, intelligible, correct and in routine use?
  - YES → Is there evidence that the individual took an unacceptable risk?
    - NO → Advise individual to consult Trade Union Representative. Consider • Corrective training • Improved supervision • Occupational Health referral • Reasonable adjustment to duties. **Highlight any System Failures identified**
  - NO → Substitution Test
- NO → Substitution Test

Substitution Test

Would another individual coming from the same professional group, possessing comparable qualifications and experience, behave in the same way in similar circumstances?
- YES → System Failure
- NO → Were there any deficiencies in training, experience or supervision?
  - YES → System Failure
  - NO → Is there evidence that the individual took an unacceptable risk?

Were there significant mitigating circumstances?
- YES → System Failure
- NO → Consult NCCA or relevant regulatory body. Advise individual to consult Trade Union Representative. Consider • Referral to disciplinary/regulatory body • Reasonable adjustment to duties • Occupational Health referral • Suspension. **Highlight any System Failures identified**

System Failure
Review system

Source: Adapted from Meadows, Baker, and Butler (2005).
Note: NCCA = National Commission for Certifying Agencies.

conduct, this type of error should be tracked closely to watch for additional incidents.

Human error, the third type of error, is the most common type recognized in healthcare. Here, the error is a product of the system's design and outputs. Complex work environments and processes drive the choices humans make. In these cases, the leaders are responsible for responding in a way that ensures that changes are made in the system. Because they can rule out that the person acted in an intentional or negligent way, for example by using an incident decision tree (exhibit 31.1), the response is to fix the system (Meadows, Baker, and Butler 2005).

The value of applying just culture principles in highly reliable organizations is that they encourage transparency and reporting as well as help identify individuals who may be putting patients at risk. Most people come into work every day planning to do the best they can. A failure to address noncompliance or risky behaviors decreases the credibility of the leadership in regard to supporting patient safety.

CHAPTER 32

Training: A Corporate Responsibility

MOST HEALTHCARE OBSERVERS note that physicians and nurses in the US healthcare system lack adequate training in safety science, high-reliability organization practices, and process design. After all, clinicians are not taught safety science or the characteristics of high reliability in medical or nursing school, nor are they trained in how to design an efficient and safe process. This deficit leaves the healthcare system with a workforce that is missing an entire body of knowledge, and gaining that knowledge represents the most obvious solution to the ongoing safety crisis. Once the necessary skills have been learned and internal processes redesigned to be safe and efficient, much of that crisis will likely be addressed.

But that body of knowledge, including a vast number of tools, tactics, and processes, takes commitment and dedicated training time to learn so that a safe healthcare environment is created. For example, exhibit 32.1 lists the typical topics presented during the authors' four-and-a-half-day workshop, HRO Academy™. Even for such an extensive course, the list of new learning required to make organizations safe is not inclusive.

Exhibit 32.1: HRO Academy™ Curriculum

DAY ONE

- Our Nation's Patient Safety Crisis
- What the Public Can See—Your Public Performance Data
- The Financial Impact of Poor Quality & Safety
- What You Need to Know about High Reliability Design—The Basics+
- Creating, Sustaining, and Nurturing a SAFETY CULTURE—What It Really Takes

DAY TWO—Safety Data, Safety Dashboards, and Safety Surveys

- Serious Safety Events—Is this all you need to measure?
- The Safety Dashboard & the Preventable Harm Index
- Safety Surveys—The Intersection of Culture and Process
  - Safety Culture Survey—Interpretation and Action Plans
  - The ISMP Survey (Institute for Safe Medication Practices)—The Gap Analysis
  - Intimidation Surveys—When to Use—How to Use—How NOT to Use

DAY THREE—Your Five-Year Safety Plan

- Setting the Baseline—Year 1 Assessment
- How Safe Do You Want to Be
- Setting Your Goals at Theoretical Perfection
- Year Two through Year Five—High Level Project Plans

DAY FOUR—Your Tool Box of Safety Tools

- 10 Common Tools Everyone Should Use
- 10 Not So Common Tools
- 10 Tools for Advanced Organizations
- 10 Tools Especially for Physicians
- 10 Tools Especially for Nurses

Source: Reprinted from HRO Academy brochure.

TRAINING AS A NATIONAL PRIORITY

Continuing medical and nursing education is required to maintain licensure, which the individual professionals are responsible for obtaining. Institutional support is sometimes provided, but more often it is lacking. In addition, continuing professional education rarely if ever includes requirements for annual training in quality and safety.

In contrast to healthcare, the aviation industry takes a structured and disciplined approach to safety training and has a large library of training courses for pilots and crew (FAA 2017a). The following excerpt from the Federal Aviation Administration demonstrates that industry's priority (FAA 2017a):

> Airlines arrange, pay for, and ensure the quality of all the safety training they require of their pilots. Shift rosters are designed so that pilots can attend required training sessions, and airlines keep a close record of when pilots attend these courses, together with their renewal dates. If pilots miss or fail any training or proficiency checks, they will face restrictions until the shortfall has been corrected. This may include losing the ability to exercise the privilege of their pilot's license.

Physicians, on the other hand, often must arrange to attend many elements of their core training, such as advanced life support courses, themselves. They are also often obliged to pay for these courses out-of-pocket because healthcare organizations have limited or nonexistent continuing medical education budgets. Furthermore, they must rearrange or swap shifts or clinical sessions with their colleagues to attend.

Making the team and the system accountable for safety training reinforces the message that safety is not, and should not be, an individual responsibility. Although considered administratively burdensome by some organizations, a strong case is to be made for requiring hospitals and health systems to maintain a detailed database of all the ongoing training competencies required of their staff; provide, or arrange and pay for, all the necessary training; and arrange shifts or rosters to facilitate attendance.

As we adopt safety practices from aviation, incorporating that industry's training practices is an obvious next step to success. This process, in turn, should be supported by a nationally vetted curriculum for minimal standards for training in (1) safety science and high reliability, (2) clinical quality improvement, and (3) process design and improvement methods such as the Toyota Production System. Completing the curriculum would be a requirement to both attain and maintain licensure. Without a formalized system and curriculum, the education of caregivers will continue to be an ineffective hit-and-miss model.

COURSE DESIGNS TO GET STARTED

This section describes two courses offered by the authors that provide the foundational elements of safety science.

Frontline Training: A Two-Hour Introduction to Patient Safety

The "Introduction to Patient Safety" course is a two-hour training designed to introduce frontline staff to basic knowledge about high-reliability design and safety science. Attendees should include every staff member in the organization and should ideally become part of new-employee orientation, annual competency programs, preceptorships, and physician onboarding workshops, among other educational activities. This basic curriculum is intended to reach every full-time-equivalent staff member in the organization, from the C-suite to the front line—no exceptions.

This live, interactive workshop uses the latest adult learning techniques, and tools can be immediately applied in everyday practice. It is best conducted as a unit-based, multidisciplinary activity. The curriculum is shown in exhibit 32.2.

Safety Specialist Training

The second course is designed to educate an organization's safety specialists. These specialists fulfill an extremely critical role by serving as the subject matter experts in safety science and high-reliability design. Physician safety specialists are the go-to safety resources in their specialty; nurse safety specialists are the experts on their units. To reach this level of expertise, safety specialists must complete an extensive curriculum that goes far beyond what they may have learned in college and postgraduate study. Exhibit 32.3 shows the curriculum for this three-day workshop in safety specialist training.

Exhibit 32.2: Summary of "Front Line Training—an Introduction to Patient Safety"

A two-hour workshop conducted as a unit-based, multidisciplinary activity that covers the following areas:

- The current state of patient safety in the United States and abroad
- An introduction to safety science
- The sharp-end model
- A review of your hospital's current safety data:
  - hospital-acquired conditions, safety culture survey scores, serious event rates
- A review of just and fair culture procedures
- A starter set of safety tools and behaviors
- Live simulation exercises using safety tools and behaviors

Exhibit 32.3: Summary of "Safety Specialist Training—SST 101"

A three-day workshop conducted as a multidisciplinary activity covering the following areas:

- The current state of patient safety in the United States and abroad
- An introduction to safety science
- The sharp-end model
- An introduction to human factors science
- Use of safety stories
- Team-based training
- Facilitated debriefing
- A review of your hospital's current safety data
  - hospital-acquired conditions, safety culture survey scores, serious event rates
- Safety culture survey
- Leadership tools and behaviors
- Safety tools and behaviors
- Techniques to escalate concerns
- A review of just and fair culture procedures
- Live simulation exercises using safety tools and behaviors

Additional Training Resources

Following is a short list of trainers and education companies the authors deem worthy of consideration to provide safety training:

- Root Inc. (www.rootinc.com)
  - "For over 25 years, global organizations have relied on Root to realize positive transformative, strategic or culture change. Through its research-driven disruptive methodologies, Root helps organizations create meaningful and lasting change. Patient Safety is one of their many offerings."
- Outcome Engenuity and David Marx (https://www.outcome-eng.com)

- "For more than two decades now, the company has advanced the concept of Just Culture and its role in the design of effective socio-technical systems."
- The Joint Commission Center for Transforming Healthcare (www.centerfortransforminghealthcare.org/hro_portal_main.aspx)
  - "At the Joint Commission Center for Transforming Healthcare, our mission is to transform health care into a high reliability industry by developing effective solutions to health care's most critical safety and quality problems [and to continue] the quest for achieving the gold standard in health care."
- Healthcare Performance Improvement (www.pressganey.com/consulting/safety-high-reliability)
  - Now a Press Ganey solution, "The official AHRQ-listed HPI Press Ganey PSO uniquely supports the HPI community with a protected forum for sharing and learning around the HPI SEC® & SSER® Patient Measurement System and event cause analysis methods."
- Institute for Healthcare Improvement and National Patient Safety Foundation (www.ihi.org/Topics/PatientSafety/Pages/default.aspx)
  - As of May 1, 2017, "IHI and the National Patient Safety Foundation (NPSF) merged into one organization, called IHI. Together, we are combining our knowledge and resources to focus and energize the patient safety agenda in order to build systems of safety across the continuum of care."

OVERCOMING INEVITABLE BARRIERS

As with all good plans, inevitably, organizations encounter some barriers in implementing safety program education. The most common barrier to training large numbers of employees relates to bringing care providers together all at once: "We can't afford to take our nurses offline for four hours. The opportunity cost is prohibitive." This objection can be silenced by referring to the business cases and statistics on the patient safety crisis included in this book. Every caregiver needs training in safety science and high-reliability principles, and the reasons are straightforward.

An additional response might be, "Yes, we can afford it, because the business case is solid. Furthermore, we don't need to take our employees offline for as long a period as you think." With the attention of the objecting leader captured, the innovative training techniques discussed in the next chapter can be shared.

CHAPTER 33

The Bottle-to-Throttle Rule

Bottle-to-throttle rules, or prohibitions against drinking and piloting an aircraft, have long been used in the aviation industry (e.g., Slaughter 2016). They are as widely known among employees and observers of airlines as drunk-driving laws are imbued in the consciousness of the general public. But in healthcare, guidelines related to impairment are not specific or rigorously applied. Indeed, they are often vague and not well known by clinicians.

Here again, we find a lesson and guidelines from aviation that may be applicable to healthcare.

THE STATISTICS

The FAA shares the following statistics in its instruction of pilots (excerpted from Salazar and Antuñano 2017):

> The majority of adverse effects produced by alcohol relate to the brain, the eyes, and the inner ear—three crucial organs to a pilot.
>
> Brain effects include impaired reaction time, reasoning, judgment, and memory. Alcohol decreases the ability of the brain to make use of oxygen.

Visual symptoms include eye muscle imbalance, which leads to double vision and difficulty focusing.

Inner ear effects include dizziness, and decreased hearing perception.

If other variables are added, such as sleep deprivation, fatigue, [or] medication use . . . the negative effects are significantly magnified.

The number of serious errors committed by pilots dramatically increases at or above concentrations of 0.04% blood alcohol. This is not to say that problems don't occur below this value. Some studies have shown decrements in pilot performance with blood alcohol concentrations as low as 0.025%.

THE DANGERS OF HANGOVERS

A hangover may be just as dangerous as alcohol intoxication. Symptoms commonly associated with a hangover are headache, dizziness, dry mouth, stuffy nose, fatigue, upset stomach, irritability, impaired judgment, and increased sensitivity to bright light.

A pilot with these symptoms is not fit to safely operate an aircraft. Even after complete elimination of all of the alcohol in the body, the undesirable effects of a hangover can last 48 to 72 hours after the last drink, with hangovers adversely influencing visuospatial skills, dexterity, managerial skills, and task completion (Wiese, Shlipak, and Browner 2000; Yesavage and Leirer 1986).

For this reason, the FAA instituted strict guidelines so that pilots do not fly when hung over. Just as the adverse effects of alcohol and hangovers are serious for pilots due to the nature of their work and the potentiating effects of altitude, physicians, nurses, and other clinical staff who practice under the influence of alcohol pose great risk to patients.

AVIATION BOTTLE-TO-THROTTLE GUIDELINES

The "General Recommendations from the FAA" are as follows (excerpted from Salazar and Antuñano 2017):

1. As a minimum, adhere to all the guidelines of Federal Aviation Regulation 91.17:
   a. 8 hours from "bottle to throttle"
   b. do not fly while under the influence of alcohol
   c. do not fly while using any drug that may adversely affect safety
2. A more conservative approach is to wait 24 hours from the last use of alcohol before flying. This is especially true if intoxication occurred or if you plan to fly IFR [under instrument flight rules]. Cold showers, drinking black coffee, or breathing 100% oxygen cannot speed up the elimination of alcohol from the body.
3. Consider the effects of a hangover. Eight hours from "bottle to throttle" does not mean you are in the best physical condition to fly, or that your blood alcohol concentration is below the legal limits.
4. Recognize the hazards of combining alcohol consumption and flying.
5. Use good judgment. Your life and the lives of your passengers are at risk if you drink and fly.

STANDARD PRACTICE IN HEALTHCARE

Following is a typical medical staff policy for the management of impaired physicians found in hospitals across the country:

> If a physician is believed to be under the influence of drugs or alcohol, the physician in question will be directed to wait

until the President of the Medical Staff, Chief Medical Officer, or designee arrives, at which time a urine drug screen and blood alcohol level will be obtained in the Emergency Department or the Associate Occupational Health Services Office. Chain of custody procedure will be followed in the collection of the specimens.

The President, Chief Medical Officer, or designee may at his/her discretion direct the physician to cease providing patient care pending the results of the testing, should the President, Chief Medical Officer, or designee determine that such action is necessary to safeguard patient care.

In such instance, the President, Chief Medical Officer, or designee will arrange for immediate alternative care for the physician's patient. Should the urine screen and/or the blood alcohol level be positive, or if it is negative and the President, Chief Medical Officer, or designee determines the physician to be otherwise psychologically and/or physically impaired, the physician in question may be immediately suspended by the President, Chief Medical Officer, or designee in order to safeguard patient care.

Although this policy is explicit in directing how to handle a medical staff member suspected of being under the influence, it does not contain statements or guidelines such as the bottle-to-throttle rule or hangover guidance issued by the FAA.

Lewis and colleagues (2011) suggest that "the practicalities of introducing an analogous rule in health care would need to be carefully considered." However, healthcare organizations would be prudent to issue more explicit rules, guidelines, or restrictions that mirror those from aviation.

Additionally, all healthcare organizations should continue to encourage employees and physicians with drug or alcohol problems to engage in counseling and rehabilitation without the threat of disciplinary action.

PART VII

BRINGING IT ALL TOGETHER

CHAPTER 34

Getting Started: A Sample Project Plan and Timeline

PATIENT SAFETY EFFORTS have experienced some remarkable advancements in the past several years. Organizations often see a 50, 70, or even 90 percent decrease in serious safety events by the end of a two-year implementation plan. But to get these results, hospitals and health systems must be deliberate and scientific at the outset in their selection of tools and tactics to implement. In addition, a well-thought-out project plan is needed to guide implementation during this critical window.

This chapter provides a project plan and a list of activities for the first year of an organization's safety program (see exhibit 34.1). This is a generic template, a starting point that the authors use themselves to develop 12-, 24-, and 36-month plans for client organizations. The latest version, included here, is the result of eight years of application and refinement.

Keep in mind that the content must be customized for each organization. Thus, the tools and tactics can be mixed and matched depending on what measures the organization has already implemented, the most common errors it experiences, or the common causes of the errors.

Exhibit 34.1: Year 1 Project Plan

MONTH	ACTIVITY
Month 1	**1. Conduct the organizational assessment of current safety HRO program/practices.**
	a. Review all errors (safety events) for past two years.
	b. Identify high-risk and high-volume error types and failure modes.
	c. Establish baseline rates for all harm events.
	2. Meet with senior executives and board.
	a. Review baseline data.
	b. Present year 1 project plan and recommendations.
Month 2	**1. Develop the patient safety dashboard.**
	a. Develop dashboard containing serious safety event rate, precursor events, HACs, safety survey information, process reliability measures, etc.
	2. Engage executive, operational, and physician leaders.
	a. Conduct leadership training in microsystem model.
	b. Conduct just culture training.
Month 3	**1. Develop and improve manager-level ownership and expertise.**
	a. Implement high-reliability units.
	b. Develop unit manager champions.
	c. Charge managers with leading unit-based incident reporting.
Month 4	**1. Identify and train safety specialists systemwide.**
	a. Train one safety specialist for each service line.
	2. Establish the organization's safety-organizing structures.
	a. Create the executive leadership safety-reporting structure.
	b. Create the physician safety leadership.

	c. Create the safety leadership team.
Month 5	**1. Initiate training and education for frontline staff in the first set of safety behaviors.**
	a. VIP: Conduct training in short blasts to avoid taking staff off the front line.
	b. Use innovative adult learning technology and techniques.
Month 6	**1. Garner each unit's commitment to implement two of the following human resources tools in the next eight months:**
	a. Daily safety rounds or huddles
	b. Cause analysis–trained staff
	c. Unit-based incident reporting
	d. Unit-based safety dashboard
	e. Situational awareness program—EWS—pediatric/medical/hospital and capacity
	f. Standardized shift handoffs
	g. Standardized transition handoffs
	h. Brief–execute–debrief in procedural areas
	i. SA: Eyes-wide-open simulations
	j. Lessons-learned program
Month 7	**1. Hardwire improved integration with risk management.**
	a. Implement a standardized RCA/ACA/CCA program.
Month 8	**1. Increase physician leadership membership and opportunities.**
	a. Develop high-reliability units for physicians to lead in the following areas:
	Early warning system
	Top-10 list
	Cause analysis

(continued)

Exhibit 34.1 (*continued*)

	Disclosure
	Brief–execute–debrief
	In situ simulation
	Resident education
Months 9–12	**1. Expand and continue ongoing training in the following areas:**
	a. Safety simulation—in situ and high fidelity
	b. High-reliability training exposure for all staff
	c. Medical education in safety expansion
	d. Staff competencies in safety throughout the organization
	e. Cause analysis competencies by service line or unit
	f. Brief–execute–debrief training and implementation
	g. Safety behaviors for new staff, repeat for longer-term staff
	h. Safety coaching and rounding development
	i. Faculty development in patient safety

Note: ACA = apparent cause analysis; CCA = common cause analysis; EWS = early warning system; HAC = hospital-acquired condition; HRO = high-reliability organization; RCA = root cause analysis; SA = situational awareness.

CHAPTER 35

The Power of the CEO[1]

Flaming enthusiasm, backed up by horse sense and persistence, is the quality that most frequently makes for success.

—Dale Carnegie

A LARGE HEALTHCARE system was well into the rollout of a high-reliability safety program. During the first year and a half, it invited several nationally respected experts to help kick off the program—John Nance, Mary Anne Hilliard, Tom Peterson, Amy Anyangu, Craig Clapper, and the authors of this book.

We noticed that some remarkable occurrences had taken place during the 18-month period. First, the system CEO attended almost all of the training sessions and guest lectures. She also immersed herself in high-reliability science—she seemed to have read every publication and resource we shared with her. In addition, she hired an expert in patient safety and learned about her organization's error rates—all of them—and was especially knowledgeable about the errors that caused patient deaths. She came to understand the true impact of the errors and the critical crossroad they presented for her organization.

As she learned more, her passion for patient safety grew, and she made some visible moves to communicate the importance of safety to the organization. Safety became her stump speech; she talked about it in every forum she attended and every meeting she chaired. Even during times of internal crisis, safety was high on her list of priorities. And as time marched on, her enthusiasm was unrelenting and her passion became infectious. After she led several discussions at board meetings, the board became strong supporters of the safety work. Then, she and the board instituted safety as one of the organization's five core values. It was a calculated move to send a clear message to the organization—"Safety is one of the most important things we will do every day; it's part of who we are; it's part of our *core*; it's part of our *values*." The end result? This organization has seen its error rates plummet.

This CEO's story is not an isolated occurrence among senior healthcare leaders. More than a dozen CEOs have made the transition to a patient safety environment as they learned about high-reliability science, including Bob Connors, MD, who later received an award from the National Patient Safety Foundation for his work in leading for safety throughout Helen DeVos Children's Hospital; Paul Bonis, former president of Spectrum Health Blodgett Hospital and Spectrum Health United Hospital, who used safety as the platform to drive United Hospital to three 100 Top Hospitals awards in consecutive years; and Bruce Hagen, past president of OhioHealth Riverside Hospital and current CEO of OhioHealth Marion General Hospital, who leveraged patient safety as one of the major initiatives that led Riverside Hospital to several 100 Top Hospitals awards.

Many other CEOs have embraced patient safety as well, and they have gladly led the charge toward achieving high reliability at their organizations. As a result, they lead high-performing hospitals or health systems that are often listed among the 100 Top Hospitals, the Healthgrades Distinguished Hospitals, and the 15 Top Health Systems. But some organizations have a leader at the helm who is silent or, worse, absent regarding matters of patient safety. Their hospital's safety performance is usually mediocre at best.

A strong, vocal CEO is a key component of top-performing organizations. And because high quality and improved safety equal lowered costs, these executives often lead the most cost-effective organizations as well.

Of course, effective safety programs also take effort, resources, and unrelenting determination. They require leadership at all levels of the organization. Patient safety begins and ends at the CEO's desk. What do the CEOs of high-reliability organizations do that distinguishes them and their organizations? The following sections explore six key CEO roles that, if embraced, can propel an organization to best-in-class safety performance and cost-effectiveness.

The CEO Leads the Safety Culture Transformation

The CEO is the leading spokesperson for the safety program and thus should be a passionate leader for improvement. He or she demonstrates that safety is the organization's top priority through an unrelenting focus on safety and high reliability in conversations and every other available forum to reinforce its importance. This leading role shall not be delegated, even in organizations that have a chief medical officer or chief quality officer in place. What the CEO chooses to endorse—in public and in private—is what gets done. If the CEO is silent on the topic of patient safety, the message to the entire organization is that safety is unimportant.

The CEO Makes Quality and Safety the Number One Strategic Priority

The CEO plays a central role in crafting the strategic plan. Safety can no longer be relegated to the bottom of the list—or worse, left off altogether. If the organization believes in providing top-level quality, an error-free environment, and a great patient experience to drive its success, as well as the success of the US healthcare system, patient safety belongs at the top of the list of strategic priorities. Growth, financial performance, physician engagement—all the other priorities can be driven by great quality and safety.

The CEO Conducts a Monthly, Systematic Review of Performance

With the entire C-suite, the CEO conducts a monthly, systematic review of progress toward fulfilling the goals of the safety plan. This review should be conducted with the same depth, rigor, and sense of accountability that characterize the monthly financial and operational reviews. Safety is now a strategic priority that is central to the business's success, so it must be managed accordingly.

The CEO Enforces Accountability in the C-Suite and Is Intolerant of Holdouts

Over recent years, even some of the best-designed and best-executed quality and safety programs have been derailed by one or more C-suite leaders. The quality and safety roles of each C-suite executive must be clearly articulated and accompanied by measurable goals. The CEO holds them accountable for performance, just as he or she does for financial and operational performance. CEOs cannot tolerate holdouts or saboteurs. If they surface, they must be confronted immediately.

The CEO Becomes Well Versed in Quality and Safety

To ensure a world-class program that drives value, the CEO must have an advanced understanding of quality and safety. A CEO who demonstrates a deep knowledge of these topics from the podium to the hallway can drive a program like no other. Hagen is a perfect example. The hospitals he has led have all ended up on the top-quality lists, and that success started with his leadership.

The CEO Ensures That Appropriate Resources Are Available

Of the hundreds of organizations that the authors have visited, fewer than 5 percent of their quality and safety departments were adequately staffed, had the correct level of expertise in place, and had the tools available that they needed to improve patient safety. One 40-hospital system averaged just two and a half full-time-equivalent staff in each hospital's quality department. In another organization, key areas of expertise were missing and staffing models were as varied as the number of hospitals. The CEO must ensure that the organization's quality infrastructure has robust staffing and that those staff members have the requisite skills to create award-winning quality and safety programs.

NOTE

1. Portions of this chapter have been adapted from Byrnes (2015c).

CHAPTER 36

The Cost Impact of Poor Patient Safety[I]

Quality and safety [are] the next frontier of cost management.

–Joseph J. Fifer, FHFMA, CPA, president and CEO, Healthcare Financial Management Association

IN THE EARLY days of quality improvement, the financial impact of better quality was hotly debated. Many leaders failed to understand this equation. That day seems to have passed, with general agreement, and sufficient evidence, emerging that quality and safety projects can reduce waste in the system, save money, add revenue, generate a competitive advantage, and add market share.

In fact, industry leaders now view quality and safety as necessary for an organization's financial survival. This belief is evident in the dialogue currently raging about the need to create "value" in healthcare, where value is defined as quality divided by cost. The Healthcare Financial Management Association (HFMA) has published several white papers and a constant stream of articles in its journal, *Healthcare Financial Management*, showing how quality can affect financial performance.

REMOVING MILLIONS IN UNNECESSARY COSTS

A review of ten case studies shows that their collective financial impact from quality and safety programs was $256,354,000—roughly one quarter of a billion dollars (Byrnes 2015b). Following are a number of examples from this review that demonstrate how safe care and enhanced outcomes lead to improved financial performance.

The Cost of Avoidable Complications

According to Hollenbeak (2011), the associated costs of just one central line–associated blood stream infection were $33,000 to $75,000 per case in adult ICUs in 2009. Multiplying the cost for one preventable complication by the large number of cases in the average hospital over 12 months equates to losses approaching millions of dollars. Now consider the positive financial impact an entire quality and safety program has when an organization targets a dozen types of preventable complications. The resulting cost savings easily move into the tens of millions.

Safety Prevents Costly Claims

Children's National Medical Center in Washington, D.C., published a case study on the outcomes of its high-reliability safety program (Hilliard et al. 2012). From the program's launch in October 2008 through December 2013, the medical center instituted changes that prevented 54 errors that would have resulted in harm to patients. The organization calculated the savings in malpractice claims alone at almost $67 million.

Complication Avoidance Improves Safety

A large integrated healthcare system assessing the savings and revenue impact of the quality program at its flagship hospital identified revenue gains of $32 million from a variety of pay-for-performance

(P4P) programs and savings of $36 million from quality and safety improvements, for a total increase of $68 million. With the average complication adding $8,000 to $10,000 to the cost of a hospitalization (Fuller et al. 2009), reductions in complications and the resulting length-of-stay decreases accounted for the majority of the savings.

Lean Processes Promote Safe, Efficient Care

One project led by a Lean improvement expert generated $6.7 million in savings, as calculated by the organization's financial analysts and confirmed by both finance and clinical leaders. The project achieved these savings by focusing on the following issues (**bold** denotes safety issues):

- On-time starts
- Throughput and room turnover
- Opened and unused supplies ($3 million)
- Preference card variation (i.e., differences from surgeon to surgeon regarding the items they request to be on hand in the operating suite for each type of surgery they perform)
- **Nonindicated imaging studies**
- **Number of stents per case**
- **Appropriateness of procedures**

Fewer Steps Equals Safer Care

The medication administration process in the above-mentioned project included an average of 125 distinct steps from the time the physician wrote an order to the moment the patient received the medication. Using a Lean improvement approach, the process was redesigned and approximately 100 steps were eliminated. That reduction represents a hundred unnecessary steps that, together, were a source of tremendous waste, extra costs, and untold risk to patients, as each step in a process is an opportunity for error.

The Addition of Revenue Through Pay for Performance

By definition, P4P and value-based purchasing programs can add revenue to an organization's bottom line. What some leaders have not grasped is that, when reimbursement for performance and value is received, quality becomes a revenue generator, and the quality and safety department loses the stigma of being just an overhead cost center. Customized P4P programs with commercial insurance companies bring several benefits, such as the ability to match the P4P goals with the organization's safety and quality priorities. And a well-executed quality and safety program can generate significant revenue as well through value-based purchasing, as demonstrated by earlier examples in this chapter.

Best-in-class quality and safety equal financial survival in today's healthcare environment. In the current period of cost-cutting, unlike other similar periods, many of the traditional cost-cutting approaches—standardizing high-cost supplies such as orthopedic implants, limiting the number of vendors, increasing the use of generic drugs, and managing labor costs, for example—have been exhausted.

When these traditional approaches are no longer available, organizations look for savings in other areas. Few organizations take advantage of the financial power of their quality programs when faced with this challenge, but this is exactly what they should do: Leverage the organization's quality and safety programs to maximize their financial impact. Certainly, this advice should not be taken to mean leaders turn their attention from the primary purpose—to improve care for patients—but rather that a significant financial impact can be seen as well, either from reducing the cost of care or by creating additional revenue. To be successful, leaders must be strategic about selecting the right projects for their quality and safety programs and measure the financial outcomes.

NOTE

1. Portions of this chapter have been adapted from Byrnes (2015c).

CHAPTER 37

What to Adopt from *The Quality Playbook*

WHY DID WE include a section on *The Quality Playbook* in a book about safety? *The Quality Playbook* was published in 2016 as a practical guide for implementing quality and safety programs (Byrnes 2015c). The authors of the present volume have used most of the tactics presented in *The Quality Playbook* to implement safety programs at their own organizations. As a bonus to readers of this book, we summarize the tools, templates, and checklists found in *The Quality Playbook*.

PART I

Part I of *The Quality Playbook* discusses what it takes to become a top-100 hospital, how errors and patient outcomes directly affect an organization's financial performance, and how quality and safety can provide a competitive advantage and grow market share.

PART II

The second section covers what components to include in a quality and safety plan, how to focus those planning efforts, and how to use techniques from finance to drive change and manage accountability.

Some key topics include the following:

- What specific elements to include in a quality and safety plan to achieve a high rating in quality measures
- How to target scarce resources to gain the greatest improvement in error rates
- How to prove to skeptics in the organization that quality and safety programs create a positive financial impact

PART III

Part III focuses on people. A great variety of topics are covered, from assembling a kitchen cabinet to building an effective physician infrastructure. They are included to show how specific, even small, activities can derail quality and safety programs as "weak links." Shoring these up improves an organization's chances for success.

This part of *The Quality Playbook* also includes a discussion of leadership dyads, whereby large quality projects are co-led by a nurse leader and physician leader. In the authors' experience, no other leadership framework works as well as dyad leadership does.

In addition, several chapters are dedicated to physician infrastructure to address the underutilization of physician leaders. Once organized, empowered, and trained, these leaders play a significant role in reducing errors.

Staffing models and skill sets for the quality and safety department are included as well, demonstrating how to make a business case for adequate staffing. Quality and safety are everyone's job, so organizing "everyone" should be a large part of the plan.

PART IV

In part IV, *The Quality Playbook* covers the most important tools and strategies that put the theory into action in a commonsense, simple, and straightforward manner. Following are some key topics:

- How to use data to drive improvement
- The best ways to align incentives and hardwire accountability
- The best strategies for engaging physicians in quality and safety
- How to sustain your gains, that is, how to keep performance in the top decile or better

PART V

In the final section, *The Quality Playbook* explores how to mobilize the board and the C-suite—two groups that can add a lot of momentum to an organization's quality and safety program. Support from and active participation by these groups are key elements of success in almost every high-performing organization. Information presented that some may not yet have considered includes the following:

- Specific roles for each C-suite executive
- Best practices for the board and a board quality and safety committee

References

Agency for Healthcare Research and Quality (AHRQ). 2014. "Team-STEPPS Fundamentals Course: Module 3. Evidence-Based: Communication." Reviewed October. www.ahrq.gov/teamstepps/instructor/fundamentals/module3/ebcommunication.html.

———. 2012. "Advancing Patient Safety: A Decade of Evidence, Design, and Implementation." Published September. www.ahrq.gov/professionals/quality-patient-safety/patient-safety-resources/resources/advancing-patient-safety/index.html.

Aiken, L. H., S. P. Clarke, D. M. Sloane, J. Sochalski, and J. H. Silber. 2002. "Hospital Nurse Staffing and Patient Mortality, Nurse Burnout, and Job Dissatisfaction." *Journal of the American Medical Association* 288 (16): 1987–93.

Ali, M., A. Osborne, R. Bethune, and A. Pullyblank. 2011. "Preoperative Surgical Briefings Do Not Delay Operating Room Start Times and Are Popular with Surgical Team Members." *Journal of Patient Safety* 7 (3): 139–43.

American Congress of Obstetricians and Gynecologists, District II (ACOG District II). 2017. *2013–16 Safe Mother Initiative*. Accessed July 19. www.acog.org/-/media/Districts/District-II/Public/SMI/v2/SMIReport05242017Final.pdf.

Anthony, K., C. Wiencek, C. Bauer, B. Daly, and M. K. Anthony. 2010. "No Interruptions Please: Impact of a No Interruption Zone on Medication Safety." *Critical Care Nursing* 30 (3): 21–29.

Aviation Safety Network (ASN). 2013. "2012 Exceptionally Safe Year for Aviation." Published January 1. http://news.aviation-safety.net/2013/01/01/2012-exceptionally-safe-year-for-aviation/.

Ayd, M. A. 2004. "A Remedy of Errors." *Hopkins Medicine*. Published spring/summer. www.hopkinsmedicine.org/hmn/s04/feature1.cfm.

Baker, D. P., R. Day, and E. Salas. 2006. "Teamwork as an Essential Component of High-Reliability Organizations." *Health Services Research* 41 (4, Pt. 2): 1576–98.

Barnsteiner, J. 2011. "Teaching the Culture of Safety." *OJIN: The Online Journal of Issues in Nursing* 16 (3): manuscript 5.

Berenholtz, S. M., T. Dorman, K. Ngo, and P. J. Pronovost. 2002. "Qualitative Review of Intensive Care Unit Quality Indicators." *Journal of Critical Care* 17 (1): 1–12.

Bethune, R., G. Sasirekha, A. Sahu, S. Cawthorn, and A. Pullyblank. 2011. "Use of Briefings and Debriefings as a Tool in Improving Team Work, Efficiency, and Communication in the Operating Theatre." *Postgraduate Medical Journal* 87 (1027): 331–34.

Bickel, J., E. R. Hughes, L. Tutterow, and L. Wood. 2015. "Leveraging Big Data Analytics to Uncover New Insights in Patient Safety." Presentation at National Patient Safety Foundation Patient Safety Congress, Austin, Texas, April 30.

Blom, L., P. Petersson, P. Hagell, and A. Westergren. 2015. "The Situation, Background, Assessment and Recommendation (SBAR) Model for Communication Between Health Care Professionals: A Clinical Intervention Pilot Study." *International Journal of Caring Sciences* 8 (3): 530–35.

Böhmer, A. B., F. Wappler, T. Tinschmann, P. Kindermann, D. Rixen, M. Bellendir, U. Schwanke, B. Bouillon, and M. U. Gerbershagen. 2012. "The Implementation of a Perioperative Checklist Increases Patients' Perioperative Safety and Staff Satisfaction." *Acta Anaesthesiologica Scandinavica* 56 (3): 332–38.

Bonabeau, E., and C. Meyer. 2001. "Swarm Intelligence: A Whole New Way to Think About Business." *Harvard Business Review* 79 (5): 106–14.

Botwinick, L., M. Bisognano, and C. Haraden. 2006. *Leadership Guide to Patient Safety*. IHI Innovation Series white paper. Cambridge, MA: Institute for Healthcare Improvement.

Boyd, M., D. Cumin, B. Lombard, J. Torrie, N. Civil, and J. Weller. 2014. "Read-Back Improves Information Transfer in Simulated Clinical Crises." *BMJ Quality & Safety* 23 (12): 989–93.

Brady, P. W., S. Muething, U. Kotagal, M. Ashby, R. Galagher, D. Hall, M. Goodfriend, C. White, T. M. Bracke, V. DeCastro, M. Geiser, J. Simon, K. M. Tucker, J. Olivea, P. H. Conway, and D. S. Wheeler. 2013. "Improving Situation Awareness to Reduce Unrecognized Clinical Deterioration and Serious Safety Events." *Pediatrics* 131 (1): e298–e308.

Brilli, R. J., R. E. McClead, W. V. Crandall, L. Stoverock, J. C. Berry, T. A. Wheeler, and J. T. Davis. 2013. "A Comprehensive Patient Safety Program Can Significantly Reduce Preventable Harm, Associated Costs, and Hospital Mortality." *Journal of Pediatrics* 163: 1638–45.

Byrnes, J. 2015a. "Great Physician Engagement Is Key to Great Quality." *Physician Leadership Journal* 2 (2): 40–42.

———. 2015b. "Just How Much Value Can We Create?" *Healthcare Financial Management* 39 (1): 82–83.

———. 2015c. *The Quality Playbook: A Guide for Healthcare Leaders*. Bozeman, MT: Second River Healthcare.

Centers for Disease Control and Prevention (CDC). 2017a. "Checklist for Prevention of Central Line Associated Blood Stream Infections." Accessed August 18. www.cdc.gov/hai/pdfs/bsi/checklist-for-CLABSI.pdf.

———. 2017b. "Mortality Data." Updated May 17. www.cdc.gov/nchs/nvss/deaths.htm.

———. 2016. "HAI Data and Statistics." Updated October 25. www.cdc.gov/hai/surveillance/index.html.

Cha, A. E. 2016. "Researchers: Medical Errors Now Third Leading Cause of Death in United States." *Washington Post*. Published May 3. www.washingtonpost.com/news/to-your-health/wp/2016/05/03/researchers-medical-errors-now-third-leading-cause-of-death-in-united-states.

Children's Hospitals' Solutions for Patient Safety. 2017. "Our Results." Accessed January 1. www.solutionsforpatientsafety.org/our-results.

Clapper, C., and K. Crea. 2010. "Common Cause Analysis." *Patient Safety and Quality Healthcare* (May/June): 30–35.

Clements, L., M. Moore, T. Tribble, and J. Blake. 2014. "Reducing Skin Breakdown in Patients Receiving Extracorporeal Membranous Oxygenation." *Nursing Clinics* 49 (1): 61–68.

Connors, Bob (president, Helen DeVos Children's Hospital), in discussion with John Byrnes, June 2017.

Council on Patient Safety in Women's Health Care. 2015. "Obstetric Hemorrhage (+AIM)." Published April. http://safehealthcareforeverywoman.org/patient-safety-bundles/obstetric-hemorrhage.

Dadiz, R., J. Weinschreider, J. Schriefer, C. Arnold, C. D. Greves, E. Crosby, H. Wang, E. Pressman, and R. Guillet. 2013. "Interdisciplinary Simulation-Based Training to Improve Delivery Room Communication." *Simulation in Healthcare* 8 (5): 279–91.

Dayton, E., and K. Henriksen. 2007. "Communication Failure: Basic Components, Contributing Factors, and the Call for Structure." *Joint Commission Journal on Quality and Patient Safety* 33 (1): 34–47.

Dekker, S. 2011. *Patient Safety: A Human Factors Approach*. Boca Raton, FL: CRC Press.

———. 2007. *Just Culture: Balancing Safety and Accountability*. Surrey, UK: Ashgate.

De Vries, E. N., H. A. Prins, R. M. Crolla, A. J. den Outer, G. van Andel, S. H. van Helden, W. S. Schlack, M. A. van Putten, D. J. Gouma, M. G. Dijkgraaf, S. M. Smorenburg, M. A. Boermeester, and SURPASS Collaborative Group. 2010. "Effect of a Comprehensive Surgical Safety System on Patient Outcomes." *New England Journal of Medicine* 363 (20): 1928–37.

De Vries, E. N., M. A. Ramrattan, S. M. Smoernburg, D. J. Gouma, and M. A. Boermeester. 2008. "The Incidence and Nature of In-Hospital Adverse Events: A Systematic Review." *Quality and Safety in Health Care* 17: 216–23.

Einav, Y., D. Gopher, I. Kara, O. Ben-Yosef, M. Lawn, N. Laufer, M. Liebergall, and Y. Donchin. 2010. "Preoperative Briefing in the Operating Room: Shared Cognition, Teamwork, and Patient Safety." *Chest* 137 (2): 443–49.

Federal Aviation Administration (FAA). 2017a. "Courses." Accessed August 8. www.faasafety.gov/gslac/alc/course_catalog.aspx.

———. 2017b. "Failure to Follow Procedures While Performing Aircraft Inspections CFR 91, 125, 135, and 121." Accessed August 18. www.faasafety.gov/files/gslac/courses/content/37/561/ffp.htm.

———. 2016. "International Aviation Safety Assessment (IASA) Program." Modified December 16. www.faa.gov/about/initiatives/iasa.

Fuller, R. L., E. C. McCullough, M. Z. Bao, and R. F. Averill. 2009. "Estimating the Costs of Potentially Preventable Hospital Acquired Complications." *Health Care Financing Review* 30 (4): 17–32.

Gamble, M. 2013. "5 Traits of High Reliability Organizations: How to Hardwire Each in Your Organization." *Becker's Hospital Review*. Published April 29. www.beckershospitalreview.com/hospital-management-administration/5-traits-of-high-reliability-organizations-how-to-hardwire-each-in-your-organization.html.

Gannon, J. 1981. *Deaf Heritage: A Narrative of Deaf America*. Silver Spring, MD: National Association of the Deaf.

Garrett, C. 2008. "The Effect of Nurse Staffing Patterns on Medical Errors and Nurse Burnout." *AORN Journal* 87 (6): 1191–92.

Gartner. 2010. "Gartner Says the World of Work Will Witness 10 Changes During the Next 10 Years." Published August 4. www.gartner.com/newsroom/id/1416513.

Gregg, M. 2013. "Creating a Culture of Improving Safety." *H&HN Daily*. Published October 24. www.hhnmag.com/articles/5793-creating-a-culture-of-improving-safety.

Greenberg, C. C., S. E. Regenbogen, D. M. Studdert, S. R. Lipsitz, S. O. Rogers, M. J. Zinner, and A. A. Gawande. 2007. "Patterns of Communication Breakdowns Resulting in Injury to Surgical Patients." *Journal of the American College of Surgeons* 204: 533–40.

Griffith, K. S. 2010. "Error Prevention in a Just Culture: Avoiding Severity Bias." *Joint Commission Perspectives* 10 (6): 7–9.

Grissinger, M. 2014. "Too Many Abandon the Second Victims of Medical Error." *Pharmacy and Therapeutics* 39 (9): 591–92.

Grout, J. 2007. *Mistake-Proofing the Design of Health Care Processes*. Agency for Healthcare Research and Quality. Published May. https://archive.ahrq.gov/professionals/quality-patient-safety/patient-safety-resources/resources/mistakeproof/mistakeproofing.pdf.

Gurses, A. P., A. A. Ozok, and P. J. Pronovost. 2012. "Time to Accelerate Integration of Human Factors and Ergonomics in Patient Safety." *BMJ Quality and Safety* 21 (4): 347–51.

Healthcare Performance Improvement. 2009. *SEC℠ & SSER℠ Patient Safety Measurement System for Healthcare*. Revised December. http://hpiresults.com/docs/PatientSafetyMeasurementSystem.pdf.

Health Foundation. 2016. *Patient Safety First: 2008 to 2010—the Campaign Review*. Site last edited December. www.patientsafetyfirst.nhs.uk/ashx/Asset.ashx?path=/Patient%20Safety%20First%20-%20the%20campaign%20review.pdf.

Helmreich, R. L., J. A. Wilhelm, J. R. Klinect, and A. C. Merritt. 2001. "Culture, Error and Crew Resource Management." In *Improving Teamwork in Organizations: Applications of Resource Management Training*, edited by E. Salas, C. A. Bowers, and E. Edens, 302–28. Mahwah, NJ: Lawrence Erlbaum Associates.

Hill, M. R., M. J. Roberts, M. L. Alderson, and T. C. Gale. 2015. "Safety Culture and the 5 Steps to Safer Surgery: An Intervention Study." *British Journal of Anaesthesiology* 114 (6): 958–62.

Hilliard, M. A., R. Sczudlo, L. Scafidi, R. Cady, A. Villard, and R. Shah. 2012. "Our Journey to Zero: Reducing Serious Safety Events by Over 70% Through High-Reliability Techniques and Workforce Engagement." *Journal of Healthcare Risk Management* 32 (2): 4–18.

Hines, S., K. Luna, J. Lofthus, M. Marquardt, and D. Stelmokas. 2008. "Becoming a High Reliability Organization: Operational Advice for Hospital Leaders." Agency for Healthcare Research and Quality. Published April. https://archive.ahrq.gov/professionals/quality-patient-safety/quality-resources/tools/hroadvice/hroadvice.pdf.

Hollenbeak, C. S. 2011. "The Cost of Catheter-Related Bloodstream Infections: Implications for the Value of Prevention." *Journal of Infusion Nursing* 34 (5): 309–13.

Horner, D. L., and M. C. Bellamy. 2012. "Care Bundles in Intensive Care." *Continuing Education in Anaesthesia, Critical Care & Pain* 12 (4): 199–202.

Institute for Healthcare Communication. 2011. "Impact of Communication in Healthcare." Published June. http://healthcarecomm.org/about-us/impact-of-communication-in-healthcare.

Institute for Healthcare Improvement Idealized Design Group (IHI) and A. Frankel. 2017. "Patient Safety Leadership WalkRounds™." Accessed July 6. www.ihi.org/resources/Pages/Tools/PatientSafetyLeadershipWalkRounds.aspx.

Institute of Medicine (IOM). 2007. *Preventing Medication Errors.* Washington, DC: National Academies Press.

———. 2000. *To Err Is Human: Building a Safer Health System.* Washington, DC: National Academies Press.

Institute for Safe Medication Practices (ISMP). 2013. "Unresolved Disrespectful Behavior in Healthcare: Practitioners Speak Up (Again)—Part 1." Published October 3. www.ismp.org/Newsletters/acutecare/showarticle.aspx?id=60.

———. 2008. "Some Red Rules Shouldn't Rule in Hospitals." *Acute Care ISMP Medication Safety Alert.* Published April 24. www.ismp.org/Newsletters/acutecare/articles/20080424.asp.

———. 2004. "Intimidation: Practitioners Speak Up About This Unresolved Problem (Part I)." *Acute Care ISMP Medication Safety Alert.* Published March 11. https://ismp.org/newsletters/acutecare/articles/20040311_2.asp.

Jain, A. L., K. C. Jones, J. Simon, and M. D. Patterson. 2015. "The Impact of a Daily Pre-operative Surgical Huddle on Interruptions, Delays, and Surgeon Satisfaction in an Orthopedic Operating Room: A Prospective Study." *Patient Safety in Surgery* 9: 8.

James, J. T. 2013. "A New, Evidence-Based Estimate of Patient Harms Associated with Hospital Care." *Journal of Patient Safety* 9 (3): 122–28.

Joint Commission. 2017. "Sentinel Event Statistics." Accessed August 18. www.jointcommission.org/Sentinel Events/Statistics.

———. 2013. "Framework for Conducting a Root Cause Analysis and Action Plan." Published March 22. www.jointcommission.org/framework_for_conducting_a_root_cause_analysis_and_action_plan.

Joint Commission Center for Transforming Healthcare. 2014. "Improving Transitions of Care: Hand-Off Communications." Updated December 22. www.centerfortransforminghealthcare.org/assets/4/6/CTH_Handoff_commun_set_final_2010.pdf.

Joint Commission Perspectives. 2012. "Joint Commission Center for Transforming Healthcare Releases Targeted Solutions Tool for Hand-Off Communications." Accessed August 8, 2017. www.jointcommission.org/assets/1/6/TST_HOC_Persp_08_12.pdf.

Jones, L. K., and S. J. O'Connor. 2016. "The Use of Red Rules in Patient Safety Culture." *Universal Journal of Management* 4 (3): 130–39.

Kessler, D., A. Cheng, and P. Mullan. 2015. "Debriefing in the Emergency Department After Clinical Events: A Practical Guide." *Annals of Emergency Medicine* 65: 690–98.

Kirkland, K. B., J. P. Briggs, S. L. Trivette, W. E. Wilkinson, and D. J. Sexton. 1999. "The Impact of Surgical-Site Infections in the 1990s: Attributable Mortality, Excess Length of Hospitalizations, and Extra Costs." *Infection Control & Hospital Epidemiology* 20 (11): 725–30.

Lawton, R., and G. Armitage. 2012. *Innovating for Patient Safety in Medicine*. Exeter, UK: Learning Matters.

Leapfrog Group. 2016. "Selecting the Right Hospital Can Reduce Your Risk of Avoidable Death by 50%, According to Analysis of Newly Updated Hospital Safety Score Grades." Press release. Published April 25. www.hospitalsafetyscore.org/about-us/newsroom/display/442022.

Levy, M. M., A. Rhodes, G. S. Phillips, S. R. Townsend, C. A. Schorr, R. Beale, T. Osborn, S. Lemeshow, J. D. Chiche, A. Artigas, and R. P. Dellinger. 2015. "Surviving Sepsis Campaign: Association Between Performance Metrics and Outcomes in a 7.5-Year Study." *Critical Care Medicine* 43 (1): 3–12.

Lewis, G., R. Vaithianathan, P. Hockey, G. Hirst, and J. Bagian. 2011. "Counterheroism, Common Knowledge, and Ergonomics: Concepts from Aviation That Could Improve Patient Safety." *Milbank Quarterly* 89 (1): 4–38.

Lingard, L., S. Espin, S. Whyte, G. Regehr, G. R. Baker, R. Reznick, J. Bohnen, B. Orser, D. Doran, and E. Grober. 2004. "Communication Failures in the Operating Room: An Observational Classification of Recurrent Types and Effects." *BMJ Quality & Safety* 13 (5): 330–34.

Lingard, L., G. Regehr, B. Orser, R. Reznick, G. R. Baker, D. Doran, S. Espin, J. Bohnen, and S. Whyte. 2008. "Evaluation of a Preoperative Checklist and Team Briefing Among Surgeons, Nurses, and Anesthesiologists to Reduce Failures in Communication." *Archives of Surgery* 143 (1): 12–18.

Loeb, J., and M. Chassin. 2013. "High Reliability in Healthcare: Getting There from Here." *Milbank Quarterly* 91 (3): 459–90.

Lucian Leape Institute, National Patient Safety Foundation. 2015. *Shining a Light: Safer Health Care Through Transparency*. Boston: National Patient Safety Foundation.

———. 2013. *Through the Eyes of the Workforce: Creating Joy, Meaning, and Safer Health Care*. Boston: National Patient Safety Foundation.

Makary, M. A., A. Mukherjee, J. B. Sexton, D. Syin, E. Goodrich, E. Hartmann, L. Rowen, C. C. Behrens, M. Marohn, and P. J. Pronovost. 2007. "Operating Room Briefings and Wrong-Site Surgery." *Journal of the American College of Surgeons* 204 (2): 236–43.

Marx, D. 2017. Outcome Engenuity home page. Accessed June 15. www.outcome-eng.com.

———. 2001. "Patient Safety and the 'Just Culture': A Primer for Health Care Executives." Published April 17. www.chpso.org/sites/main/files/file-attachments/marx_primer.pdf.

Mazzocco, K., D. B. Petitti, K. T. Fong, D. Bonacum, J. Brookey, S. Graham, R. E. Lasky, J. B. Sexton, and E. J. Thomas. 2009. "Surgical Team Behaviors and Patient Outcomes." *American Journal of Surgery* 197 (5): 678–85.

McCann, E. 2014. "Deaths by Medical Mistakes Hit Records." *Healthcare IT News*. Published July 18. www.healthcareitnews.com/news/deaths-by-medical-mistakes-hit-records.

Meadows, S., K. Baker, and J. Butler. 2005. "The Incident Decision Tree: Guidelines for Action Following Patient Safety Incidents." In *Advances in Patient Safety: From Research to Implementation*, edited by K. Henriksen, J. B. Battles, E. S. Marks, and D. Lewin. Rockville, MD: Agency for Healthcare Research and Quality.

Meister, D. 1999. *The History of Human Factors and Ergonomics*. Mahwah, NJ: Lawrence Erlbaum.

Military.com. 2017. "Military Phonetic Alphabet." Accessed January 10. www.military.com/join-armed-forces/guide-to-the-military-phonetic-alphabet.html.

Mittal, V. S., T. Sigrest, M. C. Ottolini, D. Rauch, H. Lin, B. Kit, C. P. Landrigan, and G. Flores. 2010. "Family-Centered Rounds on Pediatric Wards: A PRIS Network Survey of US and Canadian Hospitalists." *Pediatrics* 126 (1): 37–43.

Mohr, D. C., J. L. Eaton, K. M. McPhaul, and M. J. Hodgson. 2015. "Does Employee Safety Matter for Patients Too? Employee Safety Climate and Patient Safety Culture in Healthcare." Agency for Healthcare Research and Quality. Published April 22. https://psnet.ahrq.gov/resources/resource/28994/does-employee-safety-matter-for-patients-too-employee-safety-climate-and-patient-safety-culture-in-health-care.

Morath, J. 2011. "Nurses Create a Culture of Patient Safety: It Takes More Than Projects." *OJIN: The Online Journal of Issues in Nursing* 16 (3): manuscript 2.

Nance, J. J. 2012. "Patient Safety." Presentation to Sisters of Charity of Leavenworth Health System physician leadership group, Leavenworth, KS.

National Patient Safety Agency (NPSA), National Health Service. 2010. *Five Steps to Safer Surgery*. Published December. www.nrls.npsa.nhs.uk/EasySiteWeb/getresource.axd?AssetID=93286.

National Patient Safety Foundation (NPSF). 2015. *RCA²: Improving Root Cause Analyses and Actions to Prevent Harm*. Cambridge, MA: NPSF.

National Transportation Safety Board (NTSB). 2014. *Review of US Civil Aviation Accidents: Calendar Year 2011*. Washington, DC: NTSB.

———. 1975. "Eastern Air Lines, Inc., Douglas DC-9-31, N8984E." Published May 23. www.ntsb.gov/investigations/AccidentReports/Pages/AAR7509.aspx.

Nationwide Children's Hospital. 2017a. "Residency Programs." Accessed June 15. www.nationwidechildrens.org/general-pediatrics-residency.

———. 2017b. "Serious Safety Event Rate (SSER)." Accessed January 28. www.nationwidechildrens.org/serious-safety-event-rate-sser.

Navy BMR. 2007. "Communication Instructions: General." Published April. http://navybmr.com/study%20material/ACP%20121.pdf.

Neily, J., P. D. Mills, Y. Young-Xu, B. T. Carney, P. West, D. H. Berger, L. M. Mazzia, D. E. Paull, and J. P. Bagian. 2010. "Association Between Implementation of a Medical Team Training Program and Surgical Mortality." *Journal of the American Medical Association* 304 (15): 1693–700.

Pagano, M. P. 2016. *Health Communication for Health Care Professionals: An Applied Approach*. New York: Springer.

Perencevich, E. N., K. E. Sands, S. E. Cosgrove, E. Guadagnoli, E. Meara, and R. Platt. 2003. "Health and Economic Impact of Surgical Site Infections Diagnosed After Hospital Discharge." *Emerging Infectious Diseases* 9 (2): 196–203.

Peterson, T. H., S. F. Teman, and R. H. Connors. 2012. "A Safety Culture Transformation: Its Effects at a Children's Hospital." *Journal of Patient Safety* 8: 1–5.

Pronovost, P., D. Needham, S. Berenholtz, D. Sinopoli, H. Chu, S. Cosgrove, B. Sexton, R. Hyzy, R. Welsh, G. Roth, J. Bander, J. Kepros, and C. Goeschel. 2006. "An Intervention to Decrease Catheter-Related Bloodstream Infections in the ICU." *New England Journal of Medicine* 355 (26): 2725–32.

Putre, L. 2014. "The AHA McKesson Quest for Quality Prize Winner." *Hospitals & Health Networks*. Published August 12. www.hhnmag.com/articles/4062-the-aha-mckesson-quest-for-quality-prize-winner.

Reason, J. 1990. *Human Error*. Cambridge, UK: Cambridge University Press.

Rodak, S. 2013. "10 Most Identified Sentinel Event Root Causes." *Becker's Infection Control & Clinical Quality*. Published September 25. www.beckershospitalreview.com/quality/10-most-identified-sentinel-event-root-causes.html.

Rogowski, J. A., D. Staiger, T. Patrick, J. Horbar, M. Kenny, and E. T. Lake. 2013. "Nurse Staffing and NICU Infection Rates." *JAMA Pediatrics* 167 (5): 444–50.

Rowe, M. M., and H. Sherlock. 2005. "Stress and Verbal Abuse in Nursing: Do Burned Out Nurses Eat Their Young?" *Journal of Nursing Management* 13 (3): 242–48.

Salazar, G. J., and M. J. Antuñano. 2017. "Alcohol and Flying: A Deadly Combination." Federal Aviation Administration. Accessed July 24. www.faa.gov/pilots/safety/pilotsafetybrochures/media/alcohol.pdf.

Sammer, C. E., and B. R. James. 2011. "Patient Safety Culture: The Nursing Unit Leader's Role." *OJIN: The Online Journal of Issues in Nursing* 16 (3): manuscript 3.

Scharf, W. R. 2007. "Red Rules: An Error-Reduction Strategy in the Culture of Safety." *Focus on Patient Safety* 10 (1): 1–2.

Shekelle, P., P. Provost, R. M. Wachter, K. M. McDonald, K. Schoelles, S. M. Dy, K. Shojania, J. T. Reston, A. S. Adams, P. B. Angood, D. W. Bates, L. Bickman, P. Carayon, L. Donaldson, N. Duan, D. O. Farley, T. Greenhalgh, J. L. Haughom, E. Lake, R. Lilford, K. N. Lohr, G. S. Meyer, M. R. Miller, D. V. Neuhauser, G. Ryan, S. Saint, S. M. Shortell, D. P. Stevens, and K. Walshe. 2013. "The Top 10 Patient Safety Strategies That Can Be Encouraged for Adoption Now." *Annals of Internal Medicine* 158 (5, Pt. 2): 365–68.

Slaughter, G. 2016. "8-Hour 'Bottle to Throttle' Rule Sets Strict Alcohol Limit on Canadian Pilots." CTV News. Published July 19. www.ctv

news.ca/canada/8-hour-bottle-to-throttle-rule-sets-strict-alcohol-limit-on-canadian-pilots-1.2993775.

Spear, S. J. 2008. *Chasing the Rabbit: How Market Leaders Outdistance the Competition and How Great Companies Can Catch Up and Win.* New York: McGraw-Hill.

Stockmeier, C., and C. Clapper. 2011. "Daily Check-in for Safety: From Best Practice to Common Practice." *Patient Safety & Quality Healthcare.* Published September 27. www.psqh.com/analysis/daily-check-in-for-safety-from-best-practice-to-common-practice.

Stone, P. W., D. Braccia, and E. Larson. 2005. "Systematic Review of Economic Analysis of Healthcare Associated Infections." *American Journal of Infection Control* 33 (90): 501–9.

Surviving Sepsis Campaign. 2015. "Bundles." Revised April. www.survivingsepsis.org/Bundles/Pages/default.aspx.

University of Missouri Health System (MU Health). 2017. "The Scott Three-Tiered Interventional Model of Second Victim Support." Accessed August 18. www.muhealth.org/app/files/public/1405/Scotts_Three_Tier_Support.pdf.

Vogus, T. J., and K. M. Sutcliffe. 2007. "The Impact of Safety Organizing, Trusted Leadership, and Care Pathways on Reported Medication Errors in Hospital Nursing Units." *Medical Care* 45 (10): 997–1002.

Wachter, R. M. 2012. *Understanding Patient Safety*, 2nd ed. New York: McGraw-Hill.

Walker, I. A., S. Reshamwalla, and I. H. Wilson. 2012. "Surgical Safety Checklists: Do They Improve Outcomes?" *British Journal of Anaesthesia* 109 (1): 47–54.

Weick, K. E., and K. M. Sutcliffe. 2015. *Managing the Unexpected: Sustained Performance in a Complex World.* San Francisco: Jossey-Bass.

Weiser, T. G., S. E. Regenbogen, K. D. Thompson, A. B. Haynes, S. R. Lipsitz, W. R. Berry, and A. A. Gawande. 2008. "An Estimation of the Global Volume of Surgery: A Modeling Strategy Based on Available Data." *Lancet* 372 (9633): 139–44.

Whitmore, J. 2009. *Coaching for Performance*. London: Nicholas Brealey.

Wiese, J. G., M. G. Shlipak, and W. S. Browner. 2000. "The Alcohol Hangover." *Annals of Internal Medicine* 132 (11): 897–902.

World Health Organization (WHO). 2012. "Surgical Safety Web Map." Updated March 26. www.gis.harvard.edu/sites/default/files/surgicalsafety.jpg.

———. 2009. *WHO Guidelines for Safe Surgery 2009*. Geneva, Switzerland: WHO.

Wu, A. 2000. "Medical Error: The Second Victim." *BMJ* 320: 726–27.

Yesavage, J. A., and V. O. Leirer. 1986. "Hangover Effects on Aircraft Pilots 14 Hours After Alcohol Ingestion: A Preliminary Report." *American Journal of Psychiatry* 143 (12): 1546–50.

Ylisela, J. 2015. "Just Call Him Bob. Really." *Health Beat*. Published June 6. https://healthbeat.spectrumhealth.org/just-call-him-bob-really/.

Zajac, A. 2009. "FDA Seeks to Reduce Drug Dosage Errors." *Los Angeles Times*. Published November 5. http://articles.latimes.com/2009/nov/05/nation/na-fda-drugs5.

Ziewacz, J. E., A. F. Arriaga, A. M. Bader, W. R. Berry, L. Edmondson, J. M. Wong, S. R. Lipsitz, D. L. Hepner, S. Peyre, S. Nelson, D. J. Boorman, D. S. Smink, S. W. Ashley, and A. A. Gawande. 2011. "Crisis Checklists for the Operating Room: Development and Pilot Testing." *Journal of the American College of Surgeons* 213 (2): 212–19.

About the Authors

John Byrnes, MD, is a nationally recognized expert in healthcare quality and safety. He has more than 20 years of experience leading, designing, and implementing quality and safety programs throughout the United States and Europe. During his recent 11-year tenure as chief quality officer at Spectrum Health, Grand Rapids, Michigan, the organization received more than 100 quality awards, was ranked three times as one of the nation's top 15 health systems, and received multiple top-50 and top-100 hospital designations.

Dr. Byrnes is a popular speaker at regional and national conferences, including the annual meetings of the Healthcare Financial Management Association (HFMA) and the American College of Healthcare Executives. He is a member of the national faculty for the American Association for Physician Leadership (AAPL), serves on its board's Faculty Advisory Council, and teaches at the AAPL Institutes. He recently completed his term on the national Board of Directors for HFMA and has served on board quality committees for large hospital systems, multispecialty medical groups, integrated healthcare systems, and health plans. Dr. Byrnes is clinical associate professor at Michigan State University's College of Human Medicine.

Susan Teman, RN, CPPS, has 30 years of experience in healthcare leadership, quality, patient safety, and risk management. Currently, she is program manager for simulation at Helen DeVos Children's Hospital (HDVCH)/Spectrum Health in Grand Rapids, Michigan.

In this position, she is in charge of the management of the simulation program; the simulation laboratory; the associated technology, development, and implementation of the business plan for simulation; and the coordination of training programs among users by working with department leadership to establish high-level priorities and maximize the use of human factors integration principles. She led the safety culture transformation at HDVCH, which was subsequently recognized by the Lucian Leape Institute of the National Patient Safety Foundation and the Michigan Hospital Association. This work has been outlined in numerous publications.

Ms. Teman is a national speaker on patient safety for the Children's Hospital Association and for Solutions for Patient Safety.